My Journey Out of Narcissism: From Chaos to Clarity

Katashi Yoshimura

© **Copyright 2024 by Katashi Yoshimura - All rights reserved.**

The following book is provided below with the aim of delivering information that is as precise and dependable as possible. However, purchasing this book implies an acknowledgment that both the publisher and the author are not experts in the discussed topics, and any recommendations or suggestions contained herein are solely for entertainment purposes. It is advised that professionals be consulted as needed before acting on any endorsed actions.

This statement is considered fair and valid by both the American Bar Association and the Committee of Publishers Association, and it holds legal binding throughout the United States.

Moreover, any transmission, duplication, or reproduction of this work, including specific information, will be deemed an illegal act, regardless of whether it is done electronically or in print. This includes creating secondary or tertiary copies of the work or recorded copies, which are only allowed with the express written consent from the Publisher. All additional rights are reserved.

The information in the following pages is generally considered to be a truthful and accurate account of facts. As such, any negligence, use, or misuse of the information by the reader will result in actions falling solely under their responsibility. There are no scenarios in which the publisher or the original author can be held liable for any difficulties or damages that may occur after undertaking the information described herein.

Additionally, the information in the following pages is intended solely for informational purposes and should be considered as such. As fitting its nature, it is presented without assurance regarding its prolonged validity or interim quality. Mention of trademarks is done without written consent and should not be construed as an endorsement from the trademark holder.

TABLE OF CONTENTS

Introduction: I Was the Narcissist – The Beginning of My Transformation..................6

Part 1: Understanding the Narcissist Within

Chapter 1: Looking in the Mirror – Discovering My Narcissistic Traits..................11
Chapter 2: Breaking Down the Barriers – The Psychology of Narcissism..................15
2.1 Roots of Narcissism: How Childhood Shaped My Personality..................15
Chapter 3: Patterns of Manipulation – How I Controlled and Hurt Others..................18
3.1 Gaslighting and Deception: The Tools of Manipulation..................18
Chapter 4: Facing the Reality – The Damage I Caused..................21
4.1 Accepting Responsibility: Owning Up to My Mistakes..................24

Part 2: The Journey of Self-Recovery – Steps to Change

Chapter 5: Taking Responsibility – Admitting My Flaws and Apologizing..................29
5.1 The Power of Apology: Why Saying Sorry Matters..................32
Chapter 6: Rewiring My Mind – Therapy and Self-Reflection..................36
6.1 Finding the Right Help: My Journey Through Therapy..................40
6.2 Reflection and Growth: Journaling and Self-Analysis..................43
Chapter 7: The Power of Empathy – Learning to Feel for Others..................48
7.1 Building Emotional Intelligence: Understanding and Managing Emotions..................51
Chapter 8: Building New Habits – Replacing Manipulation with Authenticity..................56
8.1 Honest Communication: Speaking with Integrity
Chapter 9: Self-Forgiveness and Growth – Moving Beyond the Shame..................65
9.1 Embracing Vulnerability: Allowing Myself to Be Imperfect..................69

Part 3: Thriving After Narcissism – Practical Tools and New Perspectives

Chapter 10: Tools for Ongoing Change – Daily Practices and Mindfulness..................74
10.1 Morning Rituals: Setting a Positive Tone for the Day..................77
Chapter 11: Reinventing Relationships – Building Trust from Scratch..................81
11.1 Creating New Connections: Building Friendships with Authenticity..................84
11.2 Navigating Family Dynamics: Establishing Healthy Boundaries..................87
Chapter 12: From Self-Centered to Self-Aware – Creating a Purposeful Life..................92
12.1 Finding Purpose: Aligning Actions with Values..................95
Chapter 13: Helping Others Heal – Turning My Story into a Source of Strength..................100
13.1 Mentoring and Coaching: Supporting Others on Their Journey..................103
Conclusion: The Final Journal – A Narrative of Redemption and Peace..................108

Introduction: I Was the Narcissist – The Beginning of My Transformation

There was a time when I wore my confidence like armor. I was convinced that I was invincible, that my way was the only way, and that those around me should orbit my world like planets revolving around the sun. I basked in the glow of admiration, intoxicated by the power of my own charisma, believing that I deserved every ounce of attention and praise that came my way. I was driven, ambitious, and relentless. But I was also something else: a narcissist. And this is my story.

I didn't realize it at first. I thought I was just doing what everyone else did—striving to be the best, to win, to be noticed, to feel important. I believed my actions were justified, that my intentions were pure, even when they hurt others. I saw myself as the protagonist of my own epic, navigating a world filled with people who were either allies in my journey or obstacles to be overcome. I thought I was strong, resilient, capable. I thought I was the hero. I never imagined I could be the villain.

But there were signs, if I had cared to notice them. Relationships that started with a spark of excitement but quickly burned out, leaving behind the charred remains of misunderstanding and pain. Friendships that felt like battlegrounds, filled with unspoken competition and an underlying current of distrust. A family that seemed to shrink away from me, as if they were afraid of my shadow. And through it all, a constant, nagging feeling that something was missing, that there was a hole in the center of my being that could never quite be filled, no matter how much admiration I received or how many accomplishments I achieved.

It was during this tumultuous time that I began to write. I didn't know it then, but those pages would become the map of my own salvation, guiding me from the darkness toward a place of clarity. Here's one of the first entries I wrote—a window into my state of mind, my fears, my frustrations:

Diary Entry:

Today, I feel like I'm drowning in an ocean of my own thoughts. Everywhere I turn, there's a reminder of how I've hurt the people I care about most. My partner barely speaks to me anymore, my friends seem distant, and even my family feels like they're walking on eggshells around me. I want to scream, to demand why no one understands me, why I feel so alone. But deep down, I know the answer.

I've pushed everyone away. I've demanded too much, needed too much, taken too much. And now I'm left with this gnawing emptiness, this aching sense that something is fundamentally wrong with me. I used to think it was everyone else. They were the problem. They didn't appreciate me enough, didn't see my worth, didn't understand how hard I was working to be successful, to be important. But maybe... maybe it's me. Maybe I'm the one who can't see clearly. Maybe I've been blind to the damage I've been causing, too wrapped up in my own needs to notice the pain I'm spreading.

There's a part of me that wants to deny it, to blame everyone else, to keep pretending that I'm just misunderstood. But that voice is getting quieter, drowned out by a deeper, more insistent truth. I've been selfish. I've been controlling. I've been... cruel.

I don't know how to change. I don't know where to start. But I know I have to do something, anything, to make this feeling go away. To become someone better. Someone who can look in the mirror and not hate what they see. Someone who can love and be loved without fear.

This was the beginning. This was the moment when I finally admitted that something was deeply, fundamentally wrong—not with the world around me, but with myself. It was the first step on a long, painful journey of self-awareness and transformation. I had to learn to see myself for who I truly was, not who I pretended to be or wanted to be.

It wasn't a lightning bolt of realization or a sudden epiphany that changed me. It was a slow, painful process of peeling back the layers of denial and defensiveness, of looking at my actions with a critical eye and asking myself why I had done the things I had done. It was sitting with the discomfort of knowing that I had hurt people, that I had been wrong, that I had made mistakes. It was accepting that I was flawed, that I had weaknesses, that I was not perfect.

And it was realizing that this was okay. That it was okay to be imperfect, to be human, to make mistakes. That what mattered was not the mistakes I had made, but what I chose to do with them. That I could choose to learn from them, to grow, to become a better person. That I could choose to take responsibility for my actions, to make amends, to heal the wounds I had caused.

It was a humbling experience, to say the least. I had to learn to listen, really listen, to the people around me, to hear their pain and their hurt, to understand how my actions had affected them. I had to learn to put myself in their shoes, to feel their emotions, to empathize with their experiences. I had to learn to see the world not just from my own perspective, but from the perspectives of others. And in doing so, I began to see myself in a new light.

I began to see that I was not a monster, but a person who had made mistakes. I began to see that I was not beyond redemption, but capable of change. I began to see that I had the power to choose a different path, to become the person I wanted to be, not the person I had been.

And so, I began my journey of transformation. I started by seeking help, by finding a therapist who could guide me through the process of self-reflection and healing. I read books, attended workshops, and immersed myself in the study of narcissism, not just as a way to understand myself, but as a way to understand others. I began to practice mindfulness, to meditate, to journal, to find ways to connect with myself on a deeper level. I started to take small steps toward change, to make amends with the people I had hurt, to rebuild the relationships I had damaged.

It wasn't easy. There were times when I wanted to give up, when the pain felt too much to bear, when I doubted whether I could ever truly change. But I kept going, one step at a time, one day at a time, holding on to the hope that I could be better, that I could do better.

And slowly, gradually, I began to see the light. I began to feel a sense of peace, a sense of calm, a sense of connection that I had never felt before. I began to feel empathy, not just for others, but for myself. I began to see that I was worthy of love, not because of what I had done, but because of who I was. I began to see that I could be whole, that I could be healed, that I could be free.

This is my story. This is my journey out of narcissism, from chaos to clarity, from darkness to light. This is the beginning of my transformation. And I hope that by sharing my story, I can help others find their own path to healing, to self-awareness, to growth. Because if I can change, so can you. If I can heal, so can you. And if I can find my way out of the darkness, so can you.

Part 1: Understanding the Narcissist Within

Chapter 1: Looking in the Mirror – Discovering My Narcissistic Traits

The first time I saw myself for who I truly was, it felt like a punch to the gut. Up until that moment, I had always viewed myself as confident, self-assured, maybe even a bit charismatic—qualities I had long believed were my strengths. I was the type of person who walked into a room and immediately took charge, the kind who commanded attention and often got what I wanted. I was ambitious and driven, and I didn't think twice about pushing others aside to reach my goals. I thought these traits made me powerful, successful, and worthy of respect.

But the truth, I realized, was far more complicated.

It all started with a simple conversation, one that, at first, seemed like any other. I was talking to a close friend—someone I had known for years, someone who had always been a solid presence in my life. We were catching up, but I noticed something different in their tone, a hesitation I hadn't heard before. And then, it happened: they told me, gently but firmly, that they felt hurt by my behavior. That I had been dismissive of their feelings, that I often made everything about me, that I didn't seem to care about what was happening in their life.

My first reaction was defensive, of course. I wanted to argue, to tell them they were wrong, that they were being too sensitive. But then I saw the look in their eyes—pain, frustration, and a kind of resignation that struck me in a way I couldn't ignore. It was like a mirror had been held up to my face, and for the first time, I saw the reflection of someone I didn't recognize. I saw someone who had been so wrapped up in their own world, their own needs, that they hadn't stopped to consider how they were impacting those around them.

This was the moment that everything started to change.

As I sat with those words, I felt a mix of emotions: anger, confusion, guilt, and, more than anything, fear. Fear of what I might find if I looked too closely. Fear of admitting that maybe I wasn't the person I thought I was. Fear of confronting a truth that had been staring me in the face for far too long. But I knew I couldn't ignore it anymore. I knew that if I wanted to move forward, I had to start by looking in the mirror—really looking—and discovering the traits that had defined me for so long.

The first step was the hardest: admitting to myself that I might have been wrong. That the qualities I had always considered strengths—confidence, ambition, self-assuredness—might actually have been symptoms of something deeper, something darker. I started to do some research, to read about narcissism, and it was like a lightbulb went off in my head. The more I read, the more I recognized myself in those descriptions.

Narcissism, I learned, isn't just about being self-centered or arrogant. It's a complex personality trait that can manifest in many different ways: an exaggerated sense of self-importance, a need for constant admiration, a lack of empathy, an inability to handle criticism, and a tendency to exploit others to achieve one's own ends. These traits were like puzzle pieces that had always been there, scattered around my life, but I had never seen the full picture until now.

I began to notice the patterns in my behavior. The way I would dominate conversations, always steering them back to myself, my achievements, my struggles. The way I would dismiss the feelings of others, believing that my perspective was the only one that mattered. The way I would manipulate situations to my advantage, using charm or guilt or even anger to get what I wanted. And, perhaps most painfully, the way I had treated the people closest to me—not as equals, but as props in the story of my life.

I had always prided myself on being strong, unbreakable, someone who could handle anything life threw at me. But what I failed to realize was that my strength was often a mask for something else: insecurity. I was so afraid of being seen as weak or vulnerable that I built walls around myself, walls that kept others at a distance and kept me from truly connecting with them. I would lash out at the slightest criticism, seeing it as a threat to my carefully constructed image. I would deflect blame, refuse to apologize, and insist that I was always in the right.

Looking back, I can see how exhausting it must have been for those around me. To constantly walk on eggshells, to never feel like they could be honest with me, to always have to cater to my needs and desires. I see now that my defensiveness wasn't a sign of strength; it was a sign of fear. Fear of being exposed, fear of being rejected, fear of being seen for who I really was.

Another trait that stood out to me was my need for control. I had always believed that in order to be successful, I had to be in control—of my environment, of my relationships, of my emotions. I would go to great lengths to maintain this sense of control, even if it meant manipulating others or bending the truth to suit my needs. I would plan out conversations in my head, anticipate every possible reaction, and prepare my responses accordingly. I believed that if I could just stay one step ahead, I could avoid any unpleasant surprises, any feelings of uncertainty or vulnerability.

But the truth is, control is an illusion. No matter how hard we try, we can never fully control the people around us or the events that shape our lives. My need for control was really a need for safety, a way to protect myself from the unknown. But in my quest for control, I ended up creating chaos. I pushed people away, damaged relationships, and ultimately, isolated myself from the very connection I so desperately craved.

Vulnerability was something I had always associated with weakness. To be vulnerable was to be exposed, to risk being hurt, to open myself up to rejection or failure. And so, I did everything in my power to avoid it. I wore my confidence like armor, I used humor to deflect, I kept my true feelings hidden behind a mask of bravado. I believed that if I could just keep my guard up, I could protect myself from the pain of vulnerability.

But what I failed to realize was that vulnerability is not a weakness; it is a strength. It takes courage to be vulnerable, to show up as your true self, flaws and all. It takes strength to admit when you are wrong, to ask for help, to let others see you in your most unguarded moments. By avoiding vulnerability, I was also avoiding growth. I was stuck in a cycle of self-protection, never allowing myself to fully experience the beauty of connection, empathy, and authentic love.

As I began to peel back the layers of my narcissism, I was forced to confront the damage I had caused—to others and to myself. I thought about the relationships I had lost, the friendships I had strained, the loved ones I had hurt. I thought about the times I had used manipulation to get my way, the moments I had dismissed someone's feelings or belittled their experiences. I thought about all the times I had been so focused on my own needs that I had completely ignored the needs of those around me.

And I felt a deep, aching sense of regret. Regret for the pain I had caused, regret for the opportunities I had missed, regret for the years I had spent trapped in my own self-centered world. But regret, I learned, is only useful if it leads to change. It is not enough to feel sorry for the past; I had to take action to create a different future. I had to be willing to face the uncomfortable truth of my own behavior, to hold myself accountable, to make amends where I could, and to commit to a new way of being.

Looking in the mirror and discovering my narcissistic traits was not an easy process. It was painful, it was humbling, and at times, it felt like I was tearing myself apart piece by piece. But it was also liberating. For the first time in my life, I felt like I was truly seeing myself, flaws and all. I was no longer hiding behind the mask of who I thought I should be. I was beginning to understand who I truly was—and who I wanted to become.

I realized that I had a choice. I could continue down the path I was on, clinging to my old habits and behaviors, or I could choose a different way. I could choose to let go of the need for control, to embrace vulnerability, to practice empathy, and to build meaningful, authentic connections. I could choose to heal.

This chapter of my life was not about shaming myself for my past or beating myself up for my mistakes. It was about self-awareness, self-compassion, and self-growth. It was about recognizing that I had the power to change, that I could choose to be a different person, that I could rewrite my story.

And so, I began to take the first steps on that journey. I started to explore my patterns of behavior, to understand the root causes of my narcissism, to challenge my old beliefs and replace them with new ones. I sought out therapy, joined support groups, and started to read books on personal growth and healing. I reached out to the people I had hurt, offering sincere apologies and asking for their forgiveness. I started to practice mindfulness, meditation, and journaling as a way to connect with my inner self and cultivate self-awareness.

It wasn't easy, and there were days when I felt like giving up. But I knew that this was a journey worth taking. I knew that I wanted to be a better person, not just for myself, but for the people I loved. I wanted to build relationships based on trust, respect, and mutual understanding. I wanted to live a life that was meaningful, purposeful, and aligned with my values.

And so, I kept going. I kept looking in the mirror, facing the uncomfortable truths, and choosing to move forward. Because I knew that the only way to truly change was to confront my past, embrace my present, and create my future. And I was determined to do just that.

Chapter 2: Breaking Down the Barriers – The Psychology of Narcissism

When I first started peeling back the layers of my behavior, I realized that narcissism is far more than a set of habits or attitudes. It's a psychological framework that shapes how a person sees themselves and navigates their world. Understanding this meant going beyond the surface and examining the underlying psychological forces driving those behaviors. This journey took me back to my past, to the experiences that had molded my personality, and to the defenses I had built up in response to early influences.

Understanding the psychology of narcissism required me to break through barriers of denial and defensiveness. It meant being able to look into the mirror with honesty and accept that what I saw might not be what I wanted or even thought I was. This realization was one of the most challenging stages of my journey—coming to grips with the idea that my narcissistic behavior wasn't a superficial flaw that could be quickly corrected, but a complex web of thoughts, beliefs, and emotional reactions that I had woven over time.

Narcissism is much more than just arrogance or self-centeredness. It's rooted in a deep need for validation, a fragile self-esteem that constantly craves reinforcement, and a defense mechanism against feelings of inadequacy and vulnerability. To understand its dynamics, I had to take a long, hard look at how it had developed in my life and how it had affected my relationships, decisions, and ultimately, my very sense of self.

2.1 Roots of Narcissism: How Childhood Shaped My Personality

The seeds of narcissism are often planted in childhood, a critical period when the foundation of our personality is laid. Reflecting on my upbringing, I recognized how early experiences had shaped who I became. Childhood is like wet cement; it holds the impressions of everything it comes into contact with. As I looked back, I saw how those early years had left their mark on me, creating the patterns I would follow for decades.

I grew up in an environment where love felt conditional, always tethered to performance, approval, and achievement. Success was praised, but failure or weakness? Those were met with indifference, or worse, disappointment. I learned to equate my worth with external validation—to see myself as valuable only when others told me I was. It created a constant need to prove myself, to perform, to excel, not because I truly felt capable or confident, but because I feared the emptiness of what lay underneath.

In those early years, I developed an emotional armor. If I couldn't be loved for who I was, I'd create a version of myself that would be. I'd become the best, the brightest, the most charming—whatever it took to earn the affection and validation I craved. But that armor had consequences. It didn't just protect me; it kept others out. It turned relationships into transactions, where every interaction was a means to feed my need for approval. I was constantly on guard, always assessing, always looking for threats to my carefully constructed self-image.

There's a deep wound that sits at the heart of narcissism—a fear of being unseen, unloved, unimportant. As a child, I began to build defenses around that wound. I told myself that I didn't need anyone, that I was better, smarter, more capable than those around me. It was easier to believe that than to face the pain of feeling inadequate or unworthy. Over time, those defenses became rigid, and I lost sight of the fact that they were just that—defenses. I began to believe my own story, to live it out day after day.

As I dug deeper, I realized that many of these patterns weren't unique to me. They're common in people who develop narcissistic traits. The need to be seen as special, to stand out, to be above criticism or doubt—these are shields, ways of protecting a fragile sense of self from the fear of rejection, abandonment, or insignificance. As a child, I didn't know any of this. I only knew that I felt a gnawing hunger for validation, for attention, for love. And I would do whatever it took to get it.

I remember being praised for being smart, for getting good grades, for excelling in everything I did. But there was no room for failure, no space for mistakes. Whenever I stumbled, the reaction was swift—disapproval, disappointment, sometimes even withdrawal. It taught me that love and acceptance were earned, not freely given. It created a pattern where I became hyper-focused on achieving, on being perfect, on being what others wanted me to be. I became disconnected from my own needs, my own desires, and instead became fixated on what I thought would earn me love.

This is how narcissism grows—from the fertile soil of unmet needs and a fundamental fear of being unworthy. It's a defense mechanism that starts as a way to cope but becomes a prison. For me, it began in those early years, where I learned that the world was a place where you had to fight for every bit of affection, where being seen meant being perfect, and being loved meant being better than everyone else.

As I continued to explore the roots of my behavior, I realized that much of what I thought was strength was actually fear. My need to control situations, to dominate conversations, to always be right—these weren't signs of confidence but symptoms of insecurity. I was terrified of being seen as less than, of being exposed as flawed or inadequate. I had built my identity on a foundation of sand, always shifting, always unstable, because I didn't know how to be loved for just being me.

This journey into my past was not easy. It required me to confront the stories I had told myself, the narratives I had built to justify my actions. I had to look at the pain I had caused, not just to others, but to myself. The armor I had built to protect myself had also kept me isolated, disconnected, and ultimately unfulfilled. I began to see that the path to healing wasn't about reinforcing those defenses but about dismantling them—brick by brick, layer by layer.

Understanding the psychology of narcissism meant understanding that it wasn't just about me. It was about the people I had hurt, the relationships I had damaged, and the potential I had squandered. It was about realizing that my need to be seen, to be validated, to be special, was a cry for help—a cry that could only be answered by going back to the roots of where it all began and finding a way to heal from there.

Through this process, I came to see that healing was not about blaming myself or anyone else but about understanding the deeper currents that had shaped my life. It was about learning to forgive myself, not in a way that excused my behavior, but in a way that allowed me to move forward. It was about learning to love myself, not because I was perfect, but because I was human, flawed, and worthy of love just as I was.

Looking back, I can see how far I've come. The walls I built to protect myself have started to come down. I've learned to embrace vulnerability, to accept that I don't have all the answers, that I don't need to be perfect to be loved. I've started to see myself not as a collection of traits or behaviors, but as a person—whole, imperfect, and capable of growth.

And that, for me, is where the true journey began.

Chapter 3: Patterns of Manipulation – How I Controlled and Hurt Others

3.1 Gaslighting and Deception: The Tools of Manipulation

Gaslighting and deception were the bedrock of my manipulative tactics, the strategies I relied on most heavily to maintain control and keep others off balance. Gaslighting, in particular, became my go-to tool for distorting reality, both for myself and for those around me. It wasn't just about telling lies; it was about weaving a narrative so compelling that the other person began to doubt their own memory, perception, and sanity.

I would say things like, "I never said that," or "You're just remembering it wrong," whenever confronted with something I didn't want to acknowledge. It was a subtle undermining of the other person's confidence in their own reality. I knew exactly how to twist the facts, how to pick apart their statements, and how to make them feel as though they were the ones who were confused, overly sensitive, or just plain wrong. The more they questioned themselves, the more they relied on me to tell them what was real and what wasn't. It was a way to keep them dependent on me, to ensure that they would always come back to me for validation, for the "truth."

I thrived on this power, this ability to shape reality to fit my narrative. It felt like a secret weapon, something that put me a step ahead of everyone else. I could rewrite history with a single sentence, turn the tables in any argument, and make it so that I was never in the wrong. I made people question their sanity while reinforcing my own position of authority. It was intoxicating in a way, knowing that I held that kind of influence over someone else's mind.

Deception was another weapon in my arsenal. I would present myself in a way that was designed to evoke trust and sympathy, carefully crafting stories that put me in a favorable light. I became a master at telling people what they wanted to hear, making myself out to be the hero, the victim, or the misunderstood genius, depending on what the situation called for. I tailored my persona to match the needs and desires of others, all the while hiding my true intentions and emotions. I knew how to put on a mask that was irresistible, one that made people want to be around me, to care for me, to invest in me.

What I didn't see then was the corrosive effect these tactics had on the people around me—and on myself. Gaslighting and deception might have given me temporary control, but they left a trail of confusion, mistrust, and pain. The people I manipulated felt disoriented, constantly second-guessing themselves, and slowly losing their sense of self. And while I thought I was winning, I was actually becoming more isolated, more trapped in a web of lies of my own making. I couldn't trust anyone because I knew I wasn't trustworthy. Every relationship was built on a shaky foundation of half-truths and manipulation, and deep down, I knew that one wrong move could bring it all crashing down.

While gaslighting and deception were subtle, emotional blackmail was a more direct and potent form of manipulation. I wielded it with precision, knowing exactly how to use fear and guilt to bend people to my will. This tactic involved making others feel responsible for my emotions, my well-being, and even my happiness. I became skilled at turning their love, concern, and empathy into weapons against them.

I would say things like, "If you really loved me, you would do this," or "Do you have any idea how much pain you're causing me?" These statements were carefully crafted to make the other person feel as if they were somehow failing me, as if they were the cause of my suffering and therefore responsible for fixing it. I made them feel that their actions, however small or innocent, were somehow deeply harmful to me. And in doing so, I placed the burden of my emotions squarely on their shoulders.

Fear was another tool I used frequently. I would hint at consequences, both real and imagined, if someone didn't comply with my wishes. "You know what will happen if you don't do this," I'd say, leaving the threat vague enough to allow their imagination to fill in the blanks. I knew that fear could paralyze people, that it could make them more compliant, more willing to do whatever it took to avoid the imagined fallout. And I exploited that fear to maintain control, to keep them from challenging me or pushing back against my demands.

Emotional blackmail was about keeping others in a constant state of anxiety, making them feel that they were always on the edge of doing something wrong, of disappointing me, of triggering some catastrophic outcome. It was about making sure they always put my needs first, always prioritized my happiness above their own, because the alternative was too frightening or too guilt-inducing to contemplate. I thrived on their discomfort, on the way they tiptoed around me, always trying to avoid my wrath, my disappointment, or my sadness.

But as I look back, I see how damaging this tactic was, not just for them but for me as well. I was creating an environment of fear and guilt, one that stifled any real connection, any genuine emotion. People didn't stay around me because they loved me; they stayed because they were afraid of what would happen if they didn't. They didn't support me because they believed in me; they supported me because they felt guilty, because they thought they owed it to me. And in the process, I lost out on the very things I craved the most—real love, real trust, real companionship.

By using emotional blackmail, I was trying to fill a void within myself, a void that no amount of control or manipulation could ever truly satisfy. The more I demanded from others, the emptier I felt, because deep down, I knew that none of it was real. The love was forced, the loyalty coerced, the support conditional. I was creating a world where I could never truly feel secure, where I could never truly trust anyone, because everything was based on manipulation, on fear, on guilt.

Now, I understand that the control I thought I had was an illusion. It was a mask I wore to hide my own insecurities, my own fears, my own lack of self-worth. It was a way to avoid facing the real issues within myself, to keep from having to look in the mirror and confront the person I had become. And it worked—until it didn't. Until the cracks started to show, until the people I had manipulated began to pull away, until I was left alone with the reality of what I had done and who I had become.

I am learning now that real control doesn't come from manipulating others; it comes from understanding and managing myself. Real strength doesn't come from bending others to my will; it comes from facing my own fears, my own weaknesses, my own imperfections with courage and honesty. I am beginning to see that the tactics I used were not signs of strength, but of deep-seated insecurity and fear. And I am determined to change, to break free from the patterns of manipulation and control that once defined me, and to build a new life based on honesty, integrity, and real connection.

Chapter 4: Facing the Reality - The Damage I Caused

There comes a point in every journey of self-reflection when you can no longer hide from the truth. You can no longer paint over the cracks or distract yourself with the noise of your thoughts. This was the hardest part of my transformation—facing the damage I had caused. For so long, I convinced myself that my actions were justified, that my words were necessary, and that my manipulation was a means to an end. But eventually, I was forced to confront the harsh reality: I had caused real pain. I had left behind a trail of broken relationships, wounded hearts, and fractured lives.

In the beginning, the truth was unbearable. I had prided myself on being the smartest person in the room, the one who could read others like an open book, who could manipulate emotions to get what I wanted. But that pride, that ego, came at a high cost. It was as if I had been walking through life with blinders on, seeing only what I wanted to see. The people around me were reduced to mere objects, pawns in a game where I was always the master, always in control. I never considered the real, human consequences of my actions.

The realization began slowly, almost imperceptibly, like a crack in a dam. At first, it was just a nagging thought at the back of my mind—fleeting moments when I remembered a hurt look or a silence that hung heavy between words. I would push these thoughts away, tell myself they didn't matter, that those people were too sensitive or that they deserved it somehow. But the more I delved into self-reflection, the more these moments began to pile up, one on top of the other, until they formed a mountain of undeniable evidence.

There was the time I humiliated a friend in public, making a joke at their expense that cut too deep, all for a cheap laugh and the attention it would bring me. I saw the look on their face, a mix of shock and hurt, but I dismissed it, convinced that they were overreacting. I never stopped to think about how that moment might have lingered in their mind, how it might have chipped away at their confidence, made them feel small, unworthy. I was so focused on being seen as the funny, charming one that I ignored the cost to those around me.

Then there were the romantic relationships, the partners I claimed to love. I see now that my love was a twisted kind of love—one that was always conditional, always tied to what they could give me, how they could serve me, how they could make me feel important. I would shower them with affection and praise one moment and then withdraw it all the next if they dared to challenge me or set a boundary. I made them feel like they were walking on eggshells, always afraid of saying the wrong thing, doing the wrong thing. I manipulated their emotions, played on their fears and insecurities, all to keep them in my orbit, to ensure that they would never leave me, never abandon me.

I think of one partner in particular—a kind, gentle soul who only ever wanted to love me. I see now how I twisted that love, how I took their kindness and used it against them. I remember the day they finally left, the tears in their eyes as they told me they couldn't do it anymore, that they felt like they were losing themselves. At the time, I was angry, felt betrayed, convinced that they were the problem. But now, with the clarity of hindsight, I see that I was the one who pushed them away, who made it impossible for them to stay. I see how my need for control, for dominance, slowly eroded their spirit, made them doubt themselves, made them feel like they were never enough.

And it wasn't just romantic relationships that suffered. I hurt family members too—the people who had known me the longest, who had seen me grow, who had stood by me through thick and thin. I see now how I used their love and loyalty as a weapon, turning it against them whenever it suited me. I would lash out in anger, blame them for my own shortcomings, accuse them of not understanding me, of not supporting me enough. I made them feel like they were constantly walking a tightrope, never knowing when they might say or do something that would set me off.

I remember one Thanksgiving dinner when my sister tried to confront me about my behavior. She said she was worried about me, that she felt like I was pushing people away, that I was becoming more and more isolated. I exploded at her, accused her of meddling, of trying to control me, of not knowing anything about my life. I remember the hurt in her eyes, the way she shrank back, the tears that silently fell down her cheeks. I told myself she deserved it, that she had crossed a line, but now I see that she was only trying to reach out, to help me, to be a sister to me.

The damage wasn't always loud or dramatic; sometimes, it was quiet and insidious. It was the friendships that faded away, the phone calls that stopped coming, the invitations that were no longer extended. It was the people who gradually distanced themselves, who stopped making an effort, who chose to protect themselves from my unpredictable moods, my cutting words, my relentless need for attention. I would tell myself that I didn't need them anyway, that I was better off alone, but now I see that I was the one who drove them away, who made it impossible for them to stay.

But perhaps the greatest damage was to myself. In my quest for control, for validation, for power, I lost sight of who I was. I became so consumed by my own narrative, my own need to be right, to be important, that I forgot what it meant to be truly human. I forgot what it meant to connect with others, to be vulnerable, to be real. I built walls around myself, walls that kept others out but also kept me trapped inside, isolated, lonely, and afraid.

Facing this reality was like standing before a mirror that showed every flaw, every mistake, every moment of cruelty. It was like seeing myself for the first time, stripped of all the defenses, all the excuses, all the justifications. It was painful, excruciating even, but it was also necessary. Because without facing this truth, without acknowledging the damage I had caused, there could be no real change, no real healing.

I had to accept that I was the villain in many people's stories. I had to come to terms with the fact that I was not the hero I had always imagined myself to be, but rather the source of pain, confusion, and heartbreak. I had to let go of the idea that I was always right, always justified, always the victim. I had to accept that I had been wrong, deeply wrong, and that my actions had real, lasting consequences.

This realization didn't come all at once. It was a slow, painful process, filled with moments of denial, anger, and self-pity. There were days when I wanted to run away from it all, to retreat back into the comforting lie that I was the one who had been wronged, that I was the one who deserved sympathy and understanding. But the more I resisted, the more I realized that I couldn't move forward without first facing the reality of my past.

I began to see that the damage I caused wasn't just a series of isolated incidents, but a pattern, a way of being that permeated every aspect of my life. I saw how my need for control, for dominance, for validation, had driven me to hurt others, to push them away, to make them feel small and insignificant. I saw how I had used people as tools, as props in my own personal drama, without ever considering their feelings, their needs, their humanity.

This was the hardest truth to swallow—that I had been so blinded by my own ego, my own need to be right, that I had forgotten what it meant to truly love, to truly care, to truly connect. I had to face the fact that I had been living in a bubble of my own making, a bubble that kept me isolated, disconnected, and ultimately unfulfilled.

And so, I began the slow, painful process of making amends. I reached out to those I had hurt, those I had pushed away, those I had treated as nothing more than extensions of my own will. I apologized, not just with words, but with actions, with a commitment to change, to be better, to do better. I began to listen more, to speak less, to understand that my perspective was not the only one that mattered.

It wasn't easy. Some people were willing to forgive, to give me a second chance, while others were not. Some relationships could be mended, while others were too damaged, too broken to ever be repaired. But I learned to accept that, to accept that healing was not about getting everyone to like me again, but about becoming the kind of person who no longer needed to manipulate, to control, to hurt others to feel whole.

I learned that the real damage wasn't in the moments of conflict or confrontation, but in the quiet moments of neglect, the times when I chose my own comfort over someone else's pain, my own ego over someone else's need. I learned that healing was not a destination, but a journey, a daily commitment to be better, to do better, to live with integrity and compassion.

And so, I continue on this path, knowing that I cannot undo the past, but I can choose a different future. I can choose to face the reality of who I was, to own my mistakes, to make amends where I can, and to build a new life based on honesty, empathy, and genuine connection. I can choose to be the person I always pretended to be, not for anyone else, but for myself, for my own peace, for my own redemption.

4.1 Accepting Responsibility: Owning Up to My Mistakes

Owning up to my mistakes was like peeling away layers of armor that I had worn for years—armor that protected me from feeling the weight of my actions, the sting of guilt, and the discomfort of self-awareness. It was painful, uncomfortable, and at times felt unbearable. Yet, it was necessary. Necessary not just for my healing but for the healing of those I had wronged, hurt, and pushed away.

For years, I lived in a state of denial. I told myself that my actions were justified, that my behavior was a necessary response to the circumstances around me. I convinced myself that I was the victim—misunderstood, unappreciated, and constantly under attack. I wore my narcissism like a shield, deflecting any criticism, any attempt at holding me accountable. I had mastered the art of self-deception, constructing a narrative where I was always right, always the one who had been wronged.

The first step in accepting responsibility was recognizing that my justifications were nothing more than elaborate excuses. I had to confront the truth that my behavior was not a result of what others did to me, but rather a reflection of my own inner turmoil, my own unresolved wounds, my own insecurities and fears. This realization hit me hard. It was like standing in front of a mirror and seeing myself clearly for the first time, stripped of all the justifications and defenses I had built up over the years.

It became clear to me that my actions had been driven by a deep-seated need for control. I had hurt people not because they deserved it, but because I needed to feel powerful. I needed to feel like I was in charge, that I was the one pulling the strings. I used manipulation and deceit not as a response to others, but as a way to satisfy my own ego, my own desire to feel superior.

I had to face the reality that I had been selfish—profoundly, unrepentantly selfish. I had put my own needs, my own desires, my own fears above everything and everyone else. I had treated people not as individuals with their own thoughts, feelings, and experiences, but as tools to be used, as means to an end. This was a bitter pill to swallow. I had to admit that I had been wrong, deeply and fundamentally wrong.

The next step was to stop minimizing the impact of my actions. For so long, I had downplayed the damage I had caused. I told myself that I hadn't really hurt anyone, that people were overreacting, that they would get over it. I dismissed their feelings, their pain, as irrelevant or exaggerated. But in accepting responsibility, I had to confront the truth of what I had done. I had to acknowledge that my actions had real, lasting consequences. I had hurt people deeply, caused them real pain, and left scars that might never fully heal.

I had to understand that my behavior was not just a series of isolated incidents, but a pattern—a pattern that had affected every relationship I had ever had. I saw how my need for control, for validation, for dominance had played out again and again, in different ways, with different people, but always with the same result: pain, confusion, and broken trust. I had to face the fact that I was the common denominator, that the problem was not out there, but within me.

This realization was devastating. It felt like a punch to the gut, like the wind had been knocked out of me. I felt ashamed, deeply ashamed, in a way I had never felt before. But in that shame, I also found a strange kind of relief. For the first time, I was no longer running from the truth, no longer hiding from myself. I was facing it head-on, with all its discomfort and pain.

I began to understand that accepting responsibility wasn't just about saying the words "I'm sorry." It was about owning my mistakes fully, without reservation, without trying to shift the blame or make excuses. It was about standing in the mess I had created and saying, "Yes, this is mine. I did this." It was about acknowledging the harm I had caused, not just to others, but to myself.

I started reaching out to the people I had hurt, one by one. I knew that I couldn't undo the past, but I could at least try to make amends, to offer a genuine apology, to show that I was willing to take responsibility for my actions. I wrote letters, made phone calls, met with people face-to-face. It was one of the hardest things I've ever done. I had to face their anger, their hurt, their disappointment. I had to listen to them tell me how my actions had affected them, how I had made them feel.

There were moments when I wanted to defend myself, to explain, to justify. I wanted to say, "But you don't understand what I was going through," or "I didn't mean it that way." But I knew that these were just more excuses, more ways of avoiding the truth. So, instead, I just listened. I let their words wash over me, let their pain sink in. I let myself feel the full weight of what I had done.

Some people were willing to forgive me, to give me another chance. Others were not, and I had to accept that too. I had to accept that not everyone would be willing or able to move on, that some wounds were too deep, too fresh to be healed by a simple apology. I had to accept that I couldn't control how others would respond, that all I could do was take responsibility for my part, for my actions, for my mistakes.

Accepting responsibility also meant letting go of the need to be seen as "good." For so long, I had been obsessed with being seen as the good guy, the one who was always in the right, always justified. But now, I realized that true growth, true healing, required me to let go of that need, to embrace the fact that I had not been good, that I had hurt people, that I had been wrong. I had to be okay with being the bad guy in someone else's story, with being the one who had caused pain, who had made mistakes.

I also had to forgive myself. This was perhaps the hardest part. For so long, I had been punishing myself in subtle ways, carrying around guilt and shame like a heavy weight. I had told myself that I didn't deserve happiness, that I didn't deserve forgiveness, that I would always be defined by my mistakes. But now, I began to see that forgiveness wasn't just about others—it was also about myself. I had to forgive myself for the person I had been, for the choices I had made, for the pain I had caused.

I realized that self-forgiveness wasn't about condoning my actions or pretending they hadn't happened. It was about acknowledging them fully, accepting them as part of my story, and then choosing to move forward, to be better, to do better. It was about letting go of the shame and guilt that had held me back for so long, that had kept me stuck in a cycle of self-loathing and self-destruction.

As I began to take responsibility for my actions, I also started to see the impact of my behavior in a new light. I saw how my actions had not just hurt others, but had also hurt myself. I saw how my need for control, for validation, for dominance, had left me isolated, disconnected, and deeply unhappy. I saw how my behavior had created a cycle of pain and suffering, one that I had been trapped in for years.

I realized that by taking responsibility, I was not just making amends to others—I was also making amends to myself. I was giving myself the chance to break free from the cycle, to let go of the patterns that had kept me stuck, to create a new story, one that was based on honesty, integrity, and genuine connection.

This was not an easy process. There were days when I felt overwhelmed by guilt, by shame, by the enormity of what I had done. There were days when I wanted to give up, to go back to the old ways, to hide behind my defenses once again. But I knew that I couldn't. I knew that if I wanted to truly change, if I wanted to truly heal, I had to keep moving forward, to keep taking responsibility, no matter how hard it was.

I learned that accepting responsibility is not a one-time event, but a daily practice. It is something I have to do every day, in every moment, in every interaction. It means being honest with myself, being honest with others, being willing to admit when I'm wrong, to apologize when I've hurt someone, to make amends when I've caused harm. It means being willing to let go of my need for control, for validation, for dominance, and to embrace vulnerability, humility, and empathy.

And so, I continue on this journey, knowing that I will never be perfect, that I will never be free of mistakes, but also knowing that I can choose to take responsibility, to own my actions, to make amends, and to strive every day to be the best version of myself. I know now that true strength lies not in denying my mistakes, but in owning them, learning from them, and using them as a catalyst for growth and change.

Part 2: The Journey of Self-Recovery – Steps to Change

Chapter 5: Taking Responsibility - Admitting My Flaws and Apologizing

Taking responsibility for my actions was not an easy path to walk. It felt like stepping into a dark room, unsure of what I might find or whether I would even like what I would see. The truth, when it finally revealed itself, was a harsh reflection. Admitting my flaws was like pulling back the curtain on a performance I had been directing for years, a performance designed to keep me safe, to maintain the illusion that I was in control. But now, there was no audience to impress, no script to follow—just the raw, unfiltered reality of my mistakes.

I had spent years perfecting the art of self-deception, creating elaborate stories to justify my actions. I had convinced myself that I was always right, that my behavior was a rational response to the actions of others. Whenever someone pointed out my flaws or called me out on my behavior, I would immediately shift the blame, deflect attention, or twist the narrative to make myself look like the victim. I was a master of deflection, an expert at avoiding responsibility. But deep down, I knew I was lying to myself. I knew that the stories I told were just that—stories.

The turning point came when I could no longer ignore the truth. The weight of my actions, the hurt I had caused, became too heavy to carry. I realized that if I wanted to move forward, I needed to confront my flaws head-on. I needed to stop hiding behind excuses, stop blaming others, and start owning my mistakes. Admitting my flaws was the first step in that process. It was an acknowledgment that I was not perfect, that I had made mistakes, and that I needed to do better.

Admitting my flaws required a brutal honesty that I had never allowed myself before. I had to look at myself with fresh eyes, to see myself not as the hero of my story, but as a deeply flawed human being. I had to acknowledge the ways in which I had been selfish, manipulative, and controlling. I had to accept that I had hurt people—not just accidentally, but deliberately, in moments when I felt threatened, insecure, or out of control. I had to own up to the fact that I had used others as tools to fulfill my own needs, without considering their feelings or their humanity.

There was no room for half-measures or half-truths. I couldn't just gloss over my mistakes or minimize the impact of my actions. I had to face the full extent of the harm I had caused. This was not an easy thing to do. There were moments when I wanted to run away, to hide, to retreat back into the comfortable lies I had told myself for so long. But I knew that if I wanted to change, if I wanted to grow, I had to keep moving forward, no matter how painful it was.

Admitting my flaws also meant recognizing the patterns of behavior that had led me to this point. I had to look at the ways in which I had consistently put my needs above those of others, the ways in which I had manipulated situations to my advantage, the ways in which I had sought control and dominance at all costs. I had to acknowledge that these patterns were not accidents or coincidences—they were choices, conscious or otherwise, that I had made over and over again.

I began to see that my flaws were not just individual mistakes, but part of a larger pattern of behavior that had been present in my life for as long as I could remember. I saw how my need for validation, my fear of vulnerability, my desire for control had shaped my interactions with others. I saw how I had used people as mirrors to reflect back the image of myself that I wanted to see, rather than truly connecting with them as individuals.

This realization was both humbling and liberating. It was humbling because it forced me to confront the truth of who I was, to see myself without the rose-colored glasses I had worn for so long. It was liberating because, for the first time, I felt like I was seeing myself clearly. I was no longer hiding from my flaws or pretending they didn't exist. I was facing them head-on, and in doing so, I was beginning to take back my power.

Admitting my flaws also meant understanding that they were not fixed or immutable. I had spent so long believing that my behavior was a reflection of who I was, that my flaws were part of my identity. But now, I began to see that they were not permanent. They were habits, patterns, learned behaviors that could be changed. I realized that I had the power to choose differently, to act differently, to be different.

Once I had admitted my flaws, the next step was to apologize. I had always thought of an apology as a simple act, a few words said in passing to smooth over a conflict or to appease someone else's anger. But I came to understand that a true apology is much more than that. It is an act of humility, an acknowledgment of wrongdoing, and a commitment to change. It is a way of taking responsibility for the harm I had caused and of expressing a genuine desire to make amends.

An apology is not just about saying, "I'm sorry." It is about showing that I understand the impact of my actions, that I recognize the hurt I have caused, and that I am committed to doing better. It is about making a conscious choice to put the other person's feelings and experiences before my own, to validate their pain, and to offer a genuine expression of remorse.

I realized that apologizing was not just about the words I used, but about my attitude and my actions. It was about showing up with humility, with a willingness to listen, to understand, and to take responsibility. It was about being willing to accept whatever response I received, without defensiveness or justification. It was about recognizing that an apology was not a means to an end, but an end in itself—a way of acknowledging the past and opening the door to a different future.

As I began to apologize, I found that each apology was different. Some were met with forgiveness and understanding, while others were met with anger, hurt, or silence. I had to accept that I could not control how others would respond, that I could not demand or expect forgiveness. All I could do was offer a genuine, heartfelt apology and accept whatever came back.

There were moments when apologizing felt like walking on hot coals. I had to face the people I had hurt, to look them in the eyes, to listen to their pain. I had to hear things that were hard to hear, things that cut deep, things that I wanted to deny or defend against. But I knew that to truly apologize, I had to let go of my need to be right, my need to be understood, my need to be forgiven. I had to focus on their needs, their pain, their experience.

I came to see that apologizing was not just an act of contrition, but an act of courage. It was about facing my mistakes without flinching, about standing in the discomfort of my own wrongdoing, about acknowledging my flaws without turning away. It was about being willing to be vulnerable, to open myself up to the possibility of rejection or anger or blame, without trying to protect myself or shift the blame onto others.

I also realized that apologizing was not a one-time act, but an ongoing process. It was something I needed to do not just once, but repeatedly, in different ways, with different people. It was about recognizing that my flaws would continue to show up in my life, that I would continue to make mistakes, and that I needed to be ready to apologize, again and again, whenever it was necessary.

This process taught me a great deal about humility. I learned that humility is not about thinking less of myself, but about thinking of myself less. It is about recognizing that I am not the center of the universe, that my needs and my desires are not more important than those of others. It is about accepting that I am flawed, that I will make mistakes, and that I need to be willing to take responsibility for those mistakes, no matter how uncomfortable it might be.

Apologizing also taught me a great deal about empathy. In order to offer a genuine apology, I had to put myself in the other person's shoes, to imagine what it must have felt like to be on the receiving end of my actions. I had to listen to their stories, to hear their pain, to understand their perspective. I had to let go of my own need to be understood and focus instead on understanding them.

This was not an easy thing to do. My instinct was always to defend myself, to explain, to justify. But I realized that this was just another way of avoiding responsibility, another way of putting my own needs above those of others. I had to learn to listen without judgment, without defensiveness, without trying to make it about me. I had to learn to sit with their pain, to acknowledge it, to validate it, without trying to fix it or make it go away.

Through this process, I came to see that apologizing was not just about making things right with others, but about making things right with myself. It was about reclaiming my integrity, about living in alignment with my values, about becoming the person I wanted to be. It was about letting go of the need to be perfect, the need to be seen as good, the need to be in control. It was about embracing my flaws, my mistakes, my humanity, and using them as a catalyst for growth and change.

I began to see that the true power of an apology lies not in its ability to erase the past, but in its ability to open the door to a different future. An apology does not undo the harm that has been done, but it creates the possibility for healing, for reconciliation, for growth. It allows us to move beyond our mistakes, to learn from them, to use them as a stepping stone toward a better, more authentic version of ourselves.

And so, I continue to apologize, to take responsibility, to own my flaws. I continue to listen, to learn, to grow. I know that I will never be perfect, that I will never be free of mistakes, but I also know that I can choose, every day, to take responsibility, to admit my flaws, to apologize when I need to, and to strive to be better. This is not a destination, but a journey—one that I am committed to walking, one step at a time.

5.1 The Power of Apology: Why Saying Sorry Matters

The act of apologizing is often underestimated, seen as a mere social ritual or a necessary evil to smooth over conflicts. But for someone like me, someone who had spent years wrapped up in a narcissistic cocoon, the concept of a sincere apology was far more profound. It was not just about saying "I'm sorry." It was about unraveling years of behavior, about challenging the very core of my identity, and about learning to communicate in a language I had never spoken fluently: vulnerability.

Apologizing, for me, began with a raw acknowledgment of my flaws. The realization that I had been living a life centered on my own needs, desires, and fears was jarring. It was a confession of sorts, a coming to terms with my distorted reality where I had justified my behavior, often without ever considering its impact on others. My apologies were not just words; they were acts of dismantling the carefully constructed walls of defensiveness and denial that I had built around myself.

When I first started to understand the necessity of apologizing, it felt like an enormous surrender. Apologies, to my past self, had always seemed like a sign of weakness, a giving away of power. As a narcissist, I had become adept at deflecting blame, twisting narratives, and creating justifications that always left me blameless. I feared that admitting fault would mean losing control over how others perceived me. But I was wrong.

Through the journey of self-recovery, I began to see that a genuine apology is not a surrender; it is an act of immense courage and strength. It's a confrontation with one's ego, an honest reckoning with one's failures. To apologize meant facing the uncomfortable truth that I was flawed and imperfect. It was a process of learning to be okay with that imperfection, to see it not as a weakness but as a fundamental part of being human.

Each apology I made was a step toward reclaiming a part of myself that I had lost in the fog of narcissism. It was not just about the words; it was about embodying those words through actions that demonstrated my willingness to change. I began to understand that apologies could not be hollow gestures; they had to be backed by a commitment to different behavior, by a sincere effort to repair the damage I had caused.

In every apology, there was a story. There was the friend I had manipulated into believing they were always at fault, the partner I had emotionally neglected, the family member I had cut down with harsh words. Each person, each relationship, required a unique approach, a specific recognition of the harm I had caused. I couldn't just say, "I'm sorry" and expect things to be magically repaired. I had to understand the depths of the pain I had inflicted and show, through my words and actions, that I was committed to doing better.

One of the hardest things I faced was apologizing to those I had hurt deeply. When I first reached out to them, I felt the weight of my past actions like a heavy stone in my chest. The anxiety, the fear of rejection, the dread of hearing them say, "Your apology isn't enough," was nearly paralyzing. But I knew it was necessary. I had to own my mistakes, not just for their sake but for my own healing.

Apologizing was not just about seeking forgiveness; it was about making amends with myself. It meant facing the guilt and shame that I had suppressed for so long. I had to stop running from the consequences of my actions and start understanding the impact I had on the lives of others. I realized that each time I hurt someone, a part of me had also suffered, even if I had been too blind or too stubborn to see it.

What surprised me the most was how transformative this process was, not just for my relationships but for my sense of self. Apologizing changed the way I viewed myself in the world. It shifted my focus from self-centeredness to empathy, from defensiveness to openness. I started to see people not as tools for my validation or comfort but as individuals with their own needs, their own struggles, and their own pain. The more I apologized, the more I understood that true connection is built on trust, honesty, and mutual respect—things I had rarely given.

The act of apologizing became an act of liberation. I was no longer tied to the version of myself that needed to be right, needed to be superior, needed to be in control. I found freedom in admitting my wrongs, in letting go of the impossible standards I had set for myself and others. The apologies were not just words; they were a new way of living, a new way of seeing myself and others.

The power of apology, I learned, lies in its ability to heal, to bridge gaps, and to rebuild trust. It's not about erasing the past but about acknowledging it fully and choosing a different path moving forward. It's about accepting that we all have the capacity to cause harm, but we also have the power to choose kindness, understanding, and compassion.

I realized that apologizing didn't diminish me; it expanded me. It opened me up to new possibilities, to relationships that were more genuine and fulfilling. It taught me the value of humility, of listening, and of truly seeing the people around me. I learned that saying "I'm sorry" was not just a gesture of remorse; it was a promise to do better, to be better.

And so, I kept apologizing. Not just once, but over and over, each time I recognized a new layer of my past actions. I apologized not to be absolved but to show that I was committed to growth, that I was willing to do the work necessary to become the person I wanted to be. Each apology was a step toward self-forgiveness, a step toward a life free from the shadows of my past.

I discovered that the most important apology was the one I made to myself. For years, I had been my harshest critic, my most relentless judge. I had punished myself for my mistakes, my flaws, my failures. I had convinced myself that I was unworthy of love, of happiness, of peace. But through the act of apologizing to others, I learned to offer that same grace to myself. I learned to forgive myself for being human, for being imperfect, for being in a constant state of becoming.

Apologies, I realized, are not a final destination but a continuous journey. They are an acknowledgment that we are always in the process of growing, of learning, of healing. They are a reminder that we have the power to choose how we show up in the world, how we treat ourselves, and how we treat others. And in that choice lies the true power of saying "I'm sorry."

Chapter 6: Rewiring My Mind – Therapy and Self-Reflection

Rewiring the mind. It sounds like a daunting task, almost mechanical, like reprogramming a faulty computer. For me, it was much more profound—a dismantling of everything I had ever believed about myself, my behaviors, and my place in the world. Therapy and self-reflection were not just steps toward change; they were my lifeline. They were the tools that allowed me to unravel the tangled web of narcissism that had shaped my thoughts and actions for so many years.

The journey began with a single, terrifying step: admitting that I needed help. For someone like me, who had always prided themselves on their independence, strength, and ability to control any situation, this was a hard pill to swallow. But I knew that without help, I would remain trapped in the toxic patterns that had already caused so much pain to myself and those around me. I was stuck in a cycle, repeating the same mistakes, feeling the same emptiness, experiencing the same conflicts, and hurting the people I loved most.

My first therapy session felt like walking into a foreign land. I sat across from a stranger who was trained to see through me, who had no reason to accept my excuses or fall for my charm. There was no room for my usual tactics of manipulation, deflection, or self-aggrandizement. Here, in this small, quiet room, I was just me—raw, unfiltered, and exposed. I had to be. It was the only way forward.

The therapist asked questions that cut deeper than I expected. They weren't just interested in my story; they were dissecting it. They challenged me to confront the narratives I had constructed over the years to justify my actions. Why did I feel the need to control others? Why was validation from outside sources so critical to my sense of self-worth? Why did I constantly seek admiration, even at the cost of authenticity? I realized that therapy was not about finding comfort; it was about facing discomfort head-on.

During those early sessions, I learned the power of listening—to my therapist, to myself, to the silence that often filled the room as I struggled to find answers. I had to peel back layers of my defenses, confront uncomfortable truths, and dig into memories that I had long buried. It was like shining a flashlight into the darkest corners of my mind, where I had hidden so many fears, insecurities, and regrets. Every session felt like standing in front of a mirror, forced to see every flaw, every scar, every misstep that I had refused to acknowledge before.

One of the most painful realizations was understanding the extent of my self-deception. I had spent years convincing myself that I was in control, that my behavior was justified, that any pain I caused was a result of others' shortcomings, not my own. Therapy forced me to dismantle these beliefs and to confront the reality that my actions were often driven by deep-seated insecurities, fears of rejection, and an overwhelming need to feel significant. I began to see that my narcissistic tendencies were not a sign of strength, but a desperate attempt to protect a fragile, wounded self.

As we delved deeper, my therapist introduced me to the concept of cognitive restructuring—a technique designed to help me challenge and change the distorted thinking patterns that had defined my behavior. This was where the real work began. It wasn't just about understanding why I behaved the way I did; it was about actively changing those patterns. It was like rewiring the circuits of my brain, challenging every negative thought, every self-centered belief, every manipulative instinct.

I had to learn to recognize my cognitive distortions—the ways in which I twisted reality to fit my narrative. I saw how I magnified my own importance while minimizing the value and feelings of others. I saw how I personalized situations, always assuming that I was the center of attention, whether positively or negatively. I began to see how these distorted ways of thinking had created a prison in my mind, one where I was both the warden and the prisoner.

One of the most challenging exercises was journaling—a daily practice that became a cornerstone of my self-reflection journey. Each day, I would sit down with a notebook and confront my thoughts, emotions, and actions. I would write about the moments where I felt the urge to manipulate, to control, to seek validation. I would explore why those feelings arose, what triggers set them off, and how they connected to my past experiences and insecurities.

At first, journaling felt awkward, even pointless. But over time, it became a powerful tool for self-awareness. I began to notice patterns—how certain situations, words, or interactions would ignite old habits. I began to understand the connections between my childhood experiences, where I felt unseen or unworthy, and my adult behaviors, where I sought constant affirmation and admiration. I started to see how my actions were often a reaction to these unresolved wounds, a way of trying to fill a void that seemed bottomless.

In therapy, we worked on mindfulness practices that allowed me to stay present with my emotions, to observe them without judgment, and to understand them without being overwhelmed. Mindfulness taught me to pause, to breathe, and to respond rather than react. It was a skill that took time to develop, but it became invaluable in moments where I felt the pull of my old patterns—the urge to dominate a conversation, to prove my worth, to deflect blame. Mindfulness became a way to ground myself, to stay connected to the reality of the moment rather than getting lost in the narratives my mind had spun for so long.

My therapist also helped me explore the roots of my narcissism, guiding me through painful memories of my childhood. We discussed the dynamics of my family, the messages I received about my worth, and the ways in which I had learned to protect myself by building walls around my emotions. I began to see how my narcissistic traits had developed as a defense mechanism, a way of shielding myself from feelings of inadequacy, rejection, and abandonment. This was not about blaming my past but about understanding it, about seeing how the patterns of my childhood had shaped the patterns of my adulthood.

As I continued this journey, I learned that therapy was not a linear path; it was filled with setbacks, breakthroughs, and moments of profound doubt. There were days when I felt like I was making progress, only to find myself slipping back into old habits the next day. I had to learn to be patient with myself, to accept that healing was not about perfection but about persistence. I had to learn to forgive myself for my mistakes, to see them not as failures but as opportunities for growth.

Self-reflection, outside of therapy, became a daily practice, a commitment to honesty and introspection. I made time each day to sit with my thoughts, to examine my behaviors, to question my motives. I began to see how much of my life had been driven by fear—fear of not being enough, fear of being rejected, fear of being exposed as a fraud. I realized that my narcissistic tendencies were not about self-love but about self-preservation. They were a way of protecting a deeply insecure core, a fragile self that I had never allowed to be truly seen.

I started to work on self-compassion, a concept that felt foreign and uncomfortable. For so long, I had been my harshest critic, convinced that I needed to be perfect, to be admired, to be right. I began to see that compassion, for myself and others, was the key to real change. It was about accepting my flaws, my mistakes, and my humanity. It was about recognizing that I was not alone in my struggles, that everyone has wounds, everyone has insecurities, and everyone is on a journey of growth.

In therapy, I was encouraged to practice self-compassion by speaking to myself as I would to a friend. I had to learn to be gentle with myself, to offer kindness instead of judgment, to see my progress rather than focusing on my setbacks. It was not an easy practice; it required me to challenge years of ingrained self-criticism, but it became a crucial part of my healing.

Rewiring my mind was not just about changing my thoughts; it was about changing my relationship with myself. It was about learning to see myself with empathy, to understand that my behaviors were a product of pain and fear, and to know that I had the power to choose a different path. It was about recognizing that I was not defined by my past actions but by my willingness to grow, to change, and to become a better version of myself.

Through therapy and self-reflection, I began to build a new narrative for my life—one that was not centered on my ego but on my values, my relationships, and my desire to contribute positively to the world around me. I realized that my worth was not dependent on others' validation but on my ability to live authentically, to show up as my true self, flaws and all.

This journey of rewiring my mind has been the most challenging and rewarding experience of my life. It has taught me that true strength lies not in controlling others, but in understanding myself. It has shown me that real connection is built not on manipulation, but on vulnerability. And it has helped me see that while I may have been the narcissist, I also have the capacity for change, for empathy, and for growth.

Therapy and self-reflection were not the end of my journey; they were the beginning of a new way of living—a way of living that is more aligned with my values, more connected to the people around me, and more compassionate toward myself and others. It was the start of a transformation that continues to unfold, day by day, moment by moment, as I learn to navigate the world with a rewired mind and a renewed heart.

6.1 Finding the Right Help: My Journey Through Therapy

Finding the right help was not a straightforward process; it was a journey in itself, filled with uncertainty, skepticism, and a fair amount of fear. When I first realized I needed to seek professional help, I felt a mixture of dread and relief. Dread because I knew it meant exposing the parts of myself I had spent years hiding, and relief because I was finally admitting that I couldn't do this alone.

I had spent much of my life believing that I could handle everything on my own. I prided myself on my independence, my strength, my ability to navigate any situation. But deep down, I knew something was wrong. I could see the patterns repeating themselves, relationships deteriorating, and the same feelings of emptiness and frustration returning again and again. I knew that if I wanted to break free from the cycle of narcissism, I needed help. Real help.

The first step was acknowledging that I had a problem. This might sound simple, but it was one of the hardest things I've ever done. Narcissism thrives on denial and self-deception. For years, I had convinced myself that my behavior was justified, that any issues in my relationships were the fault of others, that I was the victim of misunderstanding or betrayal. Admitting that I was the one causing the damage meant tearing down the carefully constructed walls I had built around myself. It meant allowing myself to be vulnerable, to accept that I was flawed, that I needed guidance.

I began by researching different types of therapy, trying to understand what would be the best fit for someone like me. I read articles, watched videos, and even listened to podcasts that discussed various therapeutic approaches. Cognitive Behavioral Therapy (CBT), Dialectical Behavior Therapy (DBT), Psychodynamic Therapy—each one seemed to offer something different, and each one promised a path to healing. But I felt overwhelmed by the options. How was I supposed to know which one would work for me?

I realized that choosing the right therapy was not just about finding the right method; it was about finding the right therapist. I needed someone who would not only understand the complexities of narcissism but also have the ability to see beyond the label, to recognize the human being underneath. I wanted someone who could challenge me, hold me accountable, but also provide a safe space for me to explore my thoughts and emotions.

My first attempt was with a therapist who came highly recommended by a friend. I walked into her office with a sense of guarded optimism, hoping this would be the start of something transformative. But as we began our sessions, I quickly realized that we were not a good match. She was kind, compassionate, but she seemed hesitant to push me, to challenge me. I could sense her reluctance to confront me directly about my narcissistic traits. Instead, she focused on building rapport, creating a comfortable environment. And while that might work for some, I needed something different. I needed someone who wasn't afraid to call me out, to hold up a mirror to my face and make me see myself clearly.

After a few sessions, I decided to move on. This wasn't easy. It felt like a setback, like I was failing at therapy, which in turn triggered all sorts of defensive mechanisms. But I reminded myself that this was part of the process. Finding the right help wasn't going to be easy. It required persistence, patience, and a willingness to try again.

I continued my search, reaching out to different therapists, asking questions, setting up initial consultations. It was exhausting at times, but I knew that finding the right therapist was crucial. I had to find someone who would not only understand narcissism but who would also see me as more than just a diagnosis. I needed someone who would help me navigate the murky waters of my mind, who would guide me without judgment, who would offer insights without condemnation.

Eventually, I found a therapist who seemed like a good fit. She had experience working with clients who struggled with narcissistic tendencies, but she also had a reputation for being direct, insightful, and unapologetically honest. I was nervous as I walked into her office for the first time, unsure of what to expect. But within the first few minutes, I knew this was different. She didn't waste time on small talk; she got straight to the point, asking me why I was there, what I hoped to achieve, what I was willing to do to change.

She challenged me right from the start, pushing me to confront my behavior, my thoughts, my beliefs. She asked tough questions, questions that forced me to look at myself in ways I never had before. Why did I feel the need to control others? What was I afraid of losing if I let go of that control? Why did I crave admiration and validation so desperately? What did it say about me that I needed others to see me a certain way to feel worthy?

These questions were like arrows piercing through the armor I had built around myself. They hurt. They made me uncomfortable. But I knew this was what I needed. I needed to face the truth about myself, no matter how painful it was. I needed to understand why I had become the person I was, and how I could become someone different.

Our sessions were intense. She didn't let me off the hook, didn't allow me to hide behind excuses or rationalizations. She challenged every assumption, every justification, every lie I had told myself. She helped me see the patterns in my behavior, how my actions were driven by fear, insecurity, and a desperate need for control. She helped me understand that my narcissistic tendencies were not a sign of strength but a coping mechanism, a way of protecting myself from the pain and vulnerability I feared.

Through her guidance, I began to see the roots of my behavior, how my childhood experiences had shaped my sense of self, my relationships, my view of the world. I began to see how my need for control and validation was rooted in a deep-seated fear of rejection, of being seen as unworthy, of being exposed as a fraud. I started to understand that my narcissism was not about self-love but about self-protection. It was a way of keeping the world at a distance, of maintaining a sense of superiority to avoid feeling inadequate.

But understanding these things was just the beginning. The real work was in changing them. My therapist introduced me to different techniques and exercises designed to help me challenge my thought patterns, to break free from the cycle of narcissism. She encouraged me to practice mindfulness, to become more aware of my thoughts, my emotions, my reactions. She taught me to pause, to reflect, to question my instincts, to choose a different response.

One of the most powerful exercises was learning to identify and challenge my cognitive distortions—the ways in which I twisted reality to fit my narrative. I had to learn to recognize when I was magnifying my own importance or minimizing the value of others, when I was personalizing situations that had nothing to do with me, when I was catastrophizing or jumping to conclusions. It was hard work, and it often felt like I was fighting against my own mind. But slowly, I began to see progress. I began to catch myself in the act, to notice when I was slipping back into old patterns, to stop myself before I acted on those impulses.

Another crucial part of my therapy was learning to develop empathy, to see the world through the eyes of others. My therapist helped me understand that empathy was not just a feeling; it was a skill, something that could be cultivated and developed with practice. She encouraged me to actively listen to others, to try to understand their perspectives, their feelings, their experiences. She taught me to ask questions, to be curious, to seek understanding rather than judgment.

At first, this felt unnatural, even forced. I was so used to seeing the world through my own lens, to focusing on my needs, my desires, my feelings. But with time, I began to notice a shift. I began to feel more connected to others, more aware of their emotions, more attuned to their needs. I started to see that my actions had consequences, that my words had an impact, that my behavior could hurt or heal, depending on how I chose to act.

I also had to confront my resistance to vulnerability. For so long, I had equated vulnerability with weakness, with failure, with the risk of being hurt or rejected. But my therapist helped me see that vulnerability was not about being weak; it was about being real. It was about allowing myself to be seen, flaws and all, to connect with others on a deeper, more authentic level. She encouraged me to practice being open, to share my fears, my insecurities, my struggles. And while it was terrifying at first, I began to see the power in vulnerability. I began to see that it was the key to building genuine connections, to feeling truly understood and accepted.

Finding the right help was a journey, one that required courage, perseverance, and a willingness to face the darkest parts of myself. It was not easy, and there were moments when I wanted to give up, when I doubted whether I could change, whether I was even worth the effort. But I kept going because I knew that staying the same was no longer an option. I knew that I had to break free from the prison of my own making, that I had to find a way to live that was true to who I wanted to be, not who I had been.

Through therapy, I found the help I needed, the guidance I craved, the insights that would lead me to a new understanding of myself. I found a way to navigate the complexities of my mind, to dismantle the defenses that had kept me stuck, to build a new foundation for my life. I found a way to heal, to grow, to become the person I knew I could be. And for that, I am eternally grateful.

6.2 Reflection and Growth: Journaling and Self-Analysis

Reflection has been one of the most powerful tools on my journey toward self-awareness and healing. At the beginning of this process, it felt like I was lost in a dark, endless maze with no clear direction or purpose. My mind was a tangled web of thoughts, emotions, and unresolved memories, all tightly interwoven into a narrative that I couldn't make sense of. I knew I needed to confront the reality of my behaviors and their impact on others, but I had no idea where to start or how to navigate the murky waters of my own mind. That's when I discovered the transformative power of journaling and self-analysis.

At first, I was skeptical about the idea of journaling. It seemed like an overly simplistic activity, something akin to a high school assignment or a pastime for people who already had their lives figured out. But I had reached a point where I was willing to try anything that might help me understand myself better. So, with a blank notebook and a pen, I began to write. I had no idea what to expect, and I had no specific goals other than to let my thoughts flow freely onto the page.

The early entries in my journal were messy, disjointed, and filled with frustration and anger. I wrote about my confusion, my feelings of shame, and my deep-seated fears. I let everything spill out, unfiltered and raw. There were days when the words seemed to tumble out faster than my hand could write, and other days when I struggled to put down even a single sentence. But as I continued this practice, I began to notice patterns emerging. I began to see recurring themes in my thoughts, behaviors, and emotions—patterns that I had been blind to before.

Journaling became a mirror reflecting back at me the truths I had long avoided. It revealed the motivations behind my actions, the insecurities that fueled my need for control, and the pain I had been carrying for years without realizing it. I saw, in my own words, the ways I had justified my behavior to myself, the stories I had told to maintain my self-image, and the illusions I had constructed to protect myself from facing reality. It was a humbling and often painful process, but it was also incredibly liberating.

The act of writing forced me to slow down and truly engage with my thoughts and emotions. It created a space where I could explore my feelings without judgment or fear of reprisal. On the page, I could be honest in a way that I had never allowed myself to be with anyone else, not even myself. I could confront the uncomfortable truths about my behavior, acknowledge my flaws and mistakes, and begin to untangle the knots of shame, guilt, and denial that had kept me trapped for so long.

One of the most profound realizations that came from journaling was understanding the depth of my own self-deception. I had spent years rationalizing my actions, telling myself that my behavior was justified, that I was the victim, and that everyone else was to blame for my problems. But as I wrote and reread my entries, I could no longer ignore the inconsistencies in my narratives, the contradictions in my stories, and the lies I had told myself to avoid taking responsibility. It was as if my own words were holding up a mirror, showing me the stark reality of who I had been and what I had done.

Self-analysis became an extension of this process. It involved not just reflecting on my actions and emotions but also actively questioning them. Why did I feel the need to control others? What was I afraid of losing? What was I trying to protect or hide? What childhood experiences had shaped these behaviors, and how had I come to adopt these patterns as my own? I began to dissect my thoughts and feelings, probing deeper into the layers of my psyche to uncover the root causes of my narcissistic tendencies.

This process was far from easy. It required me to confront painful memories, to face the reality of my own shortcomings, and to accept that I was not the person I had always believed myself to be. I had to let go of the illusions I had built up around myself and embrace the uncomfortable truth of my own vulnerability. There were moments of deep sorrow and regret, times when I wanted to abandon the process altogether because it felt too overwhelming, too painful. But I knew that this was the only way forward, the only path that could lead to real change and growth.

Journaling and self-analysis also helped me identify the emotional triggers that often led me to react in narcissistic ways. I began to see how my need for validation and approval had driven me to manipulate and control those around me. I realized that my inability to handle criticism or rejection was rooted in a deep-seated fear of inadequacy, a fear that I had been carrying since childhood. I understood that my defensiveness and aggression were protective mechanisms, ways of shielding myself from the pain of feeling unworthy or unloved.

As I continued to explore these patterns, I began to see how they had played out in my relationships. I saw how I had used charm, flattery, and manipulation to draw people in, only to push them away when they got too close or challenged my self-image. I saw how I had hurt those I claimed to care about, how I had used their vulnerabilities against them, and how I had created a cycle of emotional abuse that left both them and myself scarred and damaged.

The more I wrote, the more I began to see the connections between my past experiences and my present behavior. I saw how the wounds of my childhood—feeling unseen, unheard, and unimportant—had shaped my need for constant attention and validation. I saw how the emotional neglect I had experienced had taught me to rely on manipulation and control as a means of securing love and affection. I saw how my fear of abandonment had driven me to keep people at arm's length, never allowing myself to be truly vulnerable or open.

This realization was both painful and empowering. It was painful because it forced me to confront the reality of my own brokenness, to see how my actions had been shaped by unresolved trauma and deep-seated insecurities. But it was also empowering because it gave me the clarity and insight I needed to begin making real changes. I could see, for the first time, the path I needed to take to heal and grow. I understood that I was not condemned to repeat the patterns of my past, that I had the power to choose a different way of being, a different way of relating to others.

Journaling also became a tool for cultivating self-compassion. As I wrote about my experiences, I began to develop a sense of empathy for myself. I saw how my behaviors, while harmful and destructive, were rooted in a place of deep pain and fear. I realized that I was not a monster, not inherently evil or malicious, but a person who had been hurt and who, in turn, had hurt others. This understanding allowed me to forgive myself, to begin to let go of the shame and guilt that had weighed me down for so long.

Through self-analysis, I also learned to recognize the moments when my old patterns of thinking and behaving began to resurface. I became more aware of my triggers, more mindful of my reactions, and more intentional in my choices. I learned to pause and reflect before responding, to ask myself why I was feeling a certain way, and to consider how my actions might impact others. This level of self-awareness was crucial in helping me break free from the automatic responses that had defined my behavior for so long.

One of the most surprising outcomes of my journaling practice was the realization that empathy and self-compassion are interconnected. As I developed empathy for myself, I found it easier to extend that same empathy to others. I began to see people not as obstacles or threats but as complex individuals with their own fears, insecurities, and wounds. I realized that just as I had been driven by my own pain and trauma, so too were others. This shift in perspective allowed me to approach my relationships with more kindness, patience, and understanding.

In the process of reflection and growth, I also began to set new goals for myself—goals that were focused not on external validation or control but on internal growth and authenticity. I wanted to become someone who could connect with others genuinely, who could build relationships based on trust and mutual respect, who could love and be loved without conditions or manipulation. I wanted to live a life that was honest, open, and true to my values, a life that was no longer defined by the need to protect my ego or hide my vulnerabilities.

This journey of self-reflection and growth has been a long and winding road, filled with moments of doubt, pain, and uncertainty. But it has also been a journey of profound transformation and discovery. Through journaling and self-analysis, I have come to know myself in a way that I never thought possible. I have learned to embrace my imperfections, to accept my past without letting it define me, and to move forward with a sense of purpose and clarity.

Looking back, I can see how far I have come, how much I have grown, and how much I have learned. I am no longer the person I used to be—the person who lived in fear, who sought control at all costs, who was driven by a need to prove something to the world. I am becoming someone new, someone who is learning to live with an open heart, who is willing to take risks, who is not afraid to be vulnerable, and who is committed to living a life of empathy, authenticity, and love.

Chapter 7: The Power of Empathy – Learning to Feel for Others

Empathy is often portrayed as an innate quality, something that some people naturally possess and others do not. For someone like me, who once viewed relationships through a lens of manipulation and self-interest, the concept of empathy was as foreign as it was elusive. My understanding of human interaction had been shaped by a need to control and a desire for validation, which left little room for genuine emotional connection. Learning to feel for others, to truly walk in their shoes, required me to dismantle everything I thought I knew about myself and others.

I started my journey toward empathy with a profound sense of ignorance about what it meant to connect with someone on an emotional level. My previous interactions were driven by a self-serving agenda, where understanding others was merely a strategy for manipulation. I had learned to gauge people's emotions and reactions not to relate to them but to exploit them to my advantage. This approach, while effective in maintaining control, was hollow and devoid of real human connection.

The first step in developing empathy was recognizing that it required a complete shift in my focus. Rather than being preoccupied with how others could serve my needs or reflect positively on me, I had to learn to center my attention on their experiences and feelings. This was not just about understanding their surface-level emotions but about deeply feeling their pain, joy, and everything in between. It meant that I had to let go of the need to be the center of attention and instead become genuinely interested in the experiences of those around me.

One of the most revealing exercises in my quest for empathy was engaging in active listening. I had always been an avid talker, often dominating conversations with my own stories, opinions, and desires. Listening, in my past interactions, was merely a formality—a way to appear engaged while my mind was preoccupied with preparing my next response or manipulating the situation to my benefit. Active listening, however, demanded that I suspend my own narrative and truly absorb what others were saying.

In practical terms, active listening involved giving my full attention to the speaker, making a conscious effort to understand their words, emotions, and underlying needs. It required me to be present, to avoid interrupting, and to reflect on what was being communicated. This practice was initially uncomfortable and disorienting, as it forced me to confront my own tendencies toward self-centeredness. However, as I persisted, I began to notice subtle yet profound changes in my interactions.

Through active listening, I discovered the power of validating others' emotions. In the past, I had often dismissed or invalidated the feelings of those around me, either because I couldn't relate to them or because acknowledging their feelings would undermine my control. Validation, however, is a fundamental aspect of empathy. It involves recognizing and affirming another person's emotional experience without judgment or dismissal. This practice required me to acknowledge their feelings as legitimate and significant, even if I did not fully understand or agree with them.

As I continued to practice active listening and validation, I began to experience a shift in my own emotional responses. I found myself becoming more attuned to the emotions of others, more sensitive to their needs, and more willing to offer support. This newfound ability to connect on an emotional level was both exhilarating and humbling. It allowed me to experience the richness of human relationships in a way that was previously inaccessible to me.

Another crucial aspect of developing empathy was learning to manage my own emotional responses. In the past, my interactions were often driven by a desire to protect my ego and maintain control. This meant that I was quick to react defensively or dismissively when faced with emotional vulnerability from others. To truly empathize, I had to learn to manage my own emotional triggers and reactions. This involved acknowledging my own insecurities, fears, and biases and working through them in a way that did not interfere with my ability to connect with others.

I also began to explore the concept of empathy from a cognitive perspective. Cognitive empathy involves understanding another person's perspective and recognizing their thoughts and feelings. This aspect of empathy required me to engage in conscious effort to consider how others might perceive a situation, what their motivations might be, and how their experiences might shape their responses. This cognitive approach complemented my emotional experiences, allowing me to build a more comprehensive understanding of empathy.

An essential part of this cognitive exploration was practicing perspective-taking. Perspective-taking involves putting oneself in another person's position and imagining their experiences and emotions. This practice required me to move beyond my own viewpoint and consider the world from someone else's perspective. It was a challenging exercise, as it demanded that I step outside of my own comfort zone and engage with experiences that were often unfamiliar or uncomfortable.

One exercise that proved particularly valuable in developing perspective-taking was engaging in role-playing scenarios. Role-playing allowed me to simulate different situations and practice responding from various perspectives. For example, I would write out hypothetical scenarios where I had to assume the role of someone else, experiencing their challenges, frustrations, and emotions. This exercise provided valuable insights into how different perspectives could shape behavior and reactions, deepening my understanding of empathy.

As I delved further into the practice of empathy, I also began to recognize the importance of empathy in healing relationships. Many of the relationships in my life had been damaged by my narcissistic behaviors, including manipulation, control, and a lack of emotional connection. Repairing these relationships required me to demonstrate genuine empathy, to acknowledge the harm I had caused, and to work toward rebuilding trust and understanding.

One significant aspect of this healing process was engaging in open and honest communication. I had to be willing to listen to the concerns and feelings of those I had hurt, to acknowledge their pain, and to express genuine remorse. This level of vulnerability was both daunting and essential. It required me to step outside of my comfort zone and confront the reality of my actions. Through this process, I began to experience the power of empathy not just as a concept but as a transformative force in repairing and strengthening relationships.

In addition to healing relationships, empathy also played a crucial role in my personal growth. It allowed me to develop a deeper sense of connection with others, to experience the joy and fulfillment that come from authentic relationships. It shifted my focus from self-centeredness to a more balanced perspective that valued the experiences and emotions of those around me. This shift was both liberating and enriching, allowing me to build a life that was more meaningful and fulfilling.

Developing empathy was not a quick or easy process. It required sustained effort, self-reflection, and a willingness to confront uncomfortable truths. But as I continued to practice and integrate empathy into my life, I began to experience profound changes. I became more attuned to the needs of others, more capable of building meaningful connections, and more equipped to navigate the complexities of human relationships.

Empathy is not a destination but a journey—a continuous process of learning, growing, and connecting with others on a deeper level. It is a practice that requires ongoing commitment and self-awareness. But as I look back on my journey, I am grateful for the profound impact that empathy has had on my life. It has transformed my relationships, deepened my understanding of myself and others, and allowed me to experience the richness of human connection in a way that was previously inaccessible to me.

Through the practice of empathy, I have come to appreciate the beauty of human relationships, the power of genuine connection, and the transformative potential of understanding and compassion. It has been a journey of discovery and growth, one that has reshaped my perspective and enriched my life in ways I could never have imagined.

7.1 Building Emotional Intelligence: Understanding and Managing Emotions

Emotional intelligence became the linchpin of my transformation. It's one of those terms we hear tossed around in self-help books and motivational talks, but until I began to understand its depth, I never realized how fundamental it was to changing my entire way of living. Emotional intelligence isn't just about managing emotions; it's about understanding them, recognizing them in others, and responding in a way that is compassionate, kind, and honest. For someone like me, who had spent so much of my life using emotions as weapons or shields, learning to build genuine emotional intelligence was like learning a new language.

In the beginning, I found it overwhelming to even think about emotions. I was good at hiding mine or manipulating others to suit my needs, but actually sitting with them? Understanding them? That was a foreign concept. I often felt like my emotions were dangerous—like they were wild animals waiting to pounce if I let them out of their cages. My instinct had always been to control them or to bury them under layers of intellect and rationalization. But in doing so, I had lost touch with the very essence of what it meant to be human, what it meant to connect with others in a meaningful way.

One of the first steps I had to take was to get curious about my emotions instead of fearing them. This was harder than I expected. Emotions like anger, fear, shame, and sadness had always felt like threats to my carefully constructed facade. If I admitted to feeling them, it felt like admitting weakness. But the more I tried to suppress them, the more they seeped out in destructive ways—through manipulation, control, or passive-aggressive behavior. So, I started with a simple question: What was I feeling? Not what I thought I should be feeling, not what I wanted to feel, but what was really there, beneath all the layers of pretense.

At first, it was like opening Pandora's box. I was surprised by the intensity of my emotions, by how much anger and fear I had been carrying around. There were days when it felt like too much, like I was drowning in a sea of my own unresolved feelings. But I realized that the only way out was through. I had to allow myself to feel everything I had been avoiding for so long. This wasn't an easy process. It felt like I was shedding skin, like I was peeling back layers of myself that I had kept hidden for years. I was terrified that if I allowed myself to feel these things, they would consume me, that they would prove everything I feared about myself—that I was weak, that I was broken, that I was beyond redemption.

But as I started to get comfortable with these uncomfortable emotions, I began to realize something profound: my emotions were not my enemies. They were not weaknesses or defects to be hidden away. They were messages, signals from my inner world, telling me where I needed to pay attention, where I needed to heal. Anger, for example, was often a signal that I felt violated or disrespected. Fear was a sign that I was feeling vulnerable or threatened. Sadness indicated a loss or unmet need. Instead of seeing these emotions as problems to be solved, I began to see them as clues, as keys to understanding myself better.

Building emotional intelligence required me to be honest with myself in a way I had never been before. I had to admit that I didn't have all the answers, that I was deeply flawed, and that I had hurt others out of my own pain and fear. I had to confront the parts of myself that I didn't like, the parts that felt selfish, angry, or cruel. This required a level of humility that I wasn't used to. I had always been so good at justifying my actions, at explaining away my faults or blaming them on others. But I realized that true emotional intelligence wasn't about making excuses; it was about taking responsibility.

Understanding emotions also meant learning to recognize them in real-time. This was a skill I had to develop from scratch. I began by observing my physical responses to different emotions—tightness in my chest when I was anxious, a clenching in my jaw when I was angry, a heaviness in my shoulders when I was sad. I learned to notice these physical sensations as early warning signs, clues that an emotion was beginning to surface. Instead of pushing these feelings away, I tried to name them: "I'm feeling anxious right now," or "I notice I'm getting frustrated." This simple act of naming the emotion was incredibly powerful; it created a moment of pause, a space between the feeling and my reaction.

Once I could recognize my emotions, the next step was managing them. This didn't mean suppressing or ignoring them, but rather learning how to respond in a way that was healthy and constructive. One of the most challenging aspects of this was learning to regulate my emotions without resorting to old habits like manipulation or control. When I felt a surge of anger, for instance, instead of lashing out or stonewalling, I practiced taking a few deep breaths, acknowledging the anger, and asking myself what it was trying to tell me. Was it really about the person in front of me, or was it touching on something deeper, an old wound or unmet need?

Managing emotions also meant finding healthy outlets for them. I discovered that exercise, for example, was a great way to release pent-up anger or frustration. Writing became a way to process my thoughts and feelings without dumping them on others. Talking to a therapist or a trusted friend allowed me to explore my emotions in a safe space, without fear of judgment or reprisal. These outlets helped me move through my emotions without getting stuck in them, without letting them dictate my actions.

One of the most transformative aspects of building emotional intelligence was learning to empathize with others. This was something I had struggled with my whole life. I had always seen other people's emotions as inconvenient, as obstacles to getting what I wanted. But as I began to understand my own emotions better, I realized that everyone around me had their own complex inner world, their own fears, insecurities, and needs. I began to see people not as pawns in my game, but as fellow travelers on this journey of life, each with their own struggles and dreams.

Learning to empathize meant actively listening to others, not just to their words, but to the feelings behind them. It meant being present, putting aside my own agenda, and genuinely trying to understand their experience. This was not easy for me. I was so used to dominating conversations, steering them in the direction I wanted, or using them as opportunities to show off my knowledge or wit. But I started practicing a different way of engaging. I asked open-ended questions like, "How did that make you feel?" or "What was that experience like for you?" I made a conscious effort to listen without interrupting, to let people finish their thoughts, and to reflect back what I heard to make sure I understood.

Through this practice, I began to build deeper, more authentic connections with others. I realized that empathy wasn't just about feeling sorry for someone or trying to fix their problems. It was about being fully present with them, honoring their feelings, and recognizing our shared humanity. It was about saying, "I see you, I hear you, and I'm with you," without judgment or agenda. This was a radical shift for me, and it began to transform my relationships in ways I never thought possible.

Understanding and managing emotions also required me to confront my own emotional triggers. These were the situations, people, or words that could set me off, that could send me spiraling into old patterns of anger, defensiveness, or withdrawal. I had to get honest about what triggered me and why. I realized that many of my triggers were rooted in old wounds from childhood—feelings of rejection, abandonment, or inadequacy. By understanding these triggers, I could begin to anticipate them, to prepare myself for how I might feel, and to choose a different response.

One of the most powerful tools I found for managing my triggers was mindfulness. This meant staying present, noticing my thoughts and feelings as they arose, without getting swept away by them. I practiced mindful breathing, meditation, and body scanning to help me stay grounded in the present moment. When a trigger arose, instead of reacting impulsively, I tried to observe it with curiosity: "What's coming up for me right now? What am I feeling in my body? What thoughts are going through my mind?" This created a space between the trigger and my response, allowing me to choose a different path.

As I developed these skills, I found that I was less reactive, less controlled by my emotions. I became more resilient, more able to handle difficult situations without losing my cool or retreating into old habits. I began to see that emotions, even the difficult ones, were not to be feared or avoided but embraced as part of the human experience. I learned that emotions could be my allies, guiding me toward greater self-understanding and deeper connections with others.

Building emotional intelligence was not a one-time achievement; it was an ongoing practice, a daily commitment to self-awareness and growth. There were still moments when I stumbled, when I fell back into old patterns, when I let my emotions get the best of me. But instead of beating myself up, I tried to approach these moments with compassion and curiosity. I asked myself what I could learn from these experiences, how I could do better next time. I saw each mistake not as a failure but as an opportunity for growth.

In the end, building emotional intelligence taught me that true strength lies not in control or manipulation but in vulnerability and authenticity. It taught me that it's okay to feel, to be human, to be imperfect. It taught me that the path to healing and growth is not about suppressing or denying our emotions, but about understanding them, accepting them, and using them as a bridge to connect more deeply with ourselves and others.

Chapter 8: Building New Habits – Replacing Manipulation with Authenticity

For years, manipulation was my currency in the world. It was how I got what I wanted, how I controlled my environment, how I felt powerful when I was actually afraid. Manipulation came as naturally to me as breathing, a skill honed over time through a mix of charm, persuasion, and subtle coercion. It was a strategy that served me well for a while, but eventually, it began to unravel. The realization that I was manipulating others, not only to get my way but also to feel a sense of control and superiority, became a hard truth I could no longer ignore.

The turning point came when I decided that I no longer wanted to live that way. I didn't want to be the person who viewed relationships as transactions, who saw every interaction as a game to win. I wanted to connect with others on a deeper, more genuine level. I wanted to be seen for who I truly was, not for the carefully crafted persona I had created to manipulate and deceive. The desire for authenticity began to grow stronger than the desire for control, and that was when I knew I had to change.

But change, I quickly discovered, was not just about deciding to do things differently. It was about unlearning years of ingrained habits, replacing old patterns with new, healthier ones, and confronting the discomfort that comes with doing things in a new way. It was about building new habits that would support my journey toward authenticity, habits that would allow me to engage with the world openly, honestly, and without the need for manipulation.

One of the first steps was to understand why I had relied so heavily on manipulation in the first place. I began to dig deep into my past, examining the roots of my behaviors. I realized that manipulation had become my go-to strategy because, at its core, I feared vulnerability. I feared being seen as weak, being rejected, or not being enough. Manipulation was my way of protecting myself, of maintaining a sense of control in situations where I felt powerless. It was easier to manipulate others than to confront my own fears, my own insecurities.

Acknowledging this fear was crucial. It allowed me to see that my manipulative behaviors were not just about getting what I wanted, but also about avoiding the discomfort of being vulnerable, of being real. I had to confront the reality that I had been using manipulation to fill a void, to compensate for a lack of self-worth and a fear of rejection. This realization was painful, but it was also liberating. It meant that if I wanted to change, I had to start by building habits that fostered self-acceptance, self-compassion, and a willingness to be vulnerable.

One of the new habits I had to develop was the habit of honesty. Honesty, not just with others, but with myself. For so long, I had lied to myself about who I was, about what I wanted, about why I did the things I did. I had constructed a narrative that made me the hero of my story, justifying my actions and blaming others for my shortcomings. But if I was going to replace manipulation with authenticity, I had to start by being brutally honest with myself.

I began by asking myself some hard questions: Why did I feel the need to control others? What was I afraid of losing? What was I trying to protect myself from? At first, these questions were uncomfortable, even painful. They forced me to confront parts of myself that I had long ignored or denied. But they also led me to a deeper understanding of my motivations, of the fears and insecurities that lay beneath my manipulative behaviors.

With this understanding came a newfound sense of compassion for myself. I began to see that my manipulations were not born out of malice, but out of fear and pain. I had been trying to protect myself in the only way I knew how. This realization allowed me to approach my journey toward authenticity with more gentleness, more kindness. It reminded me that I was not a bad person, just a person who had developed some bad habits in response to a difficult past.

Building new habits also required me to practice transparency in my interactions. I had to learn to speak my truth, even when it was uncomfortable, even when it meant risking rejection or conflict. I had to learn to express my needs, my desires, my feelings openly and honestly, without resorting to manipulation or coercion. This was not easy. For someone who had spent years hiding behind a facade, speaking openly and honestly felt like walking around without armor, like exposing myself to potential hurt.

I remember the first time I tried to express my needs honestly in a relationship. It felt awkward, like I was fumbling through a foreign language. I was used to dropping hints, to using passive-aggressive comments, to employing subtle tactics to get my way. But now, I was trying something new. I was stating my needs directly, without pretense or manipulation. "I feel hurt when you cancel plans at the last minute. It makes me feel like I'm not a priority. I need more consistency in our time together." Saying these words out loud felt terrifying, but it also felt freeing. It was like I was reclaiming a part of myself that I had long suppressed.

Over time, I began to see that honesty, though challenging, was a far more effective way to build trust and intimacy in my relationships. When I was open about my feelings, my fears, and my needs, I found that people responded with understanding, empathy, and a willingness to meet me halfway. I began to realize that I didn't need to manipulate others to get what I wanted; I just needed to be clear and honest about what I needed. This was a profound shift for me, one that required constant practice and vigilance.

Another important habit I had to build was the habit of active listening. For so long, I had been a passive listener, hearing only what I wanted to hear, filtering out anything that didn't align with my desires or beliefs. I realized that part of being authentic meant truly listening to others, not just to respond or to manipulate, but to understand and connect. I had to learn to listen with an open heart and an open mind, to hear not just the words, but the emotions behind them.

Active listening meant putting aside my agenda, my need to control the conversation, and focusing on the person in front of me. It meant being fully present, giving my undivided attention, and showing empathy and understanding. This was a challenging practice, especially in moments when I felt defensive or triggered. But the more I practiced, the more I began to see the value in it. I found that when I truly listened, without judgment or agenda, I was able to connect with people on a much deeper level. I began to understand their experiences, their emotions, their needs in a way I never had before.

As I continued to build these new habits, I also had to confront my old patterns. I noticed that even with the best of intentions, I would sometimes slip back into old habits of manipulation and control. I had to be vigilant, to catch myself in those moments, and to choose a different response. This required a level of self-awareness that I had not been accustomed to, but it was essential to my growth.

When I felt the urge to manipulate, I had to pause and ask myself, "What am I afraid of right now? What am I trying to protect myself from?" This pause allowed me to see the underlying fear or insecurity driving my behavior. It gave me the opportunity to choose a different path, to respond with honesty and authenticity instead of manipulation.

One of the most surprising things I discovered in this process was that authenticity didn't just benefit my relationships; it also benefited me. The more I practiced being authentic, the more at peace I felt with myself. I no longer had to carry the weight of lies or deception. I no longer had to constantly strategize or scheme to get my way. I could just be myself, flawed and imperfect, but real. This was a tremendous relief. It allowed me to relax, to breathe, to be present in the moment instead of constantly planning my next move.

Building new habits of authenticity also required me to practice self-compassion. I had to learn to forgive myself when I slipped up, to be kind to myself when I struggled. This was perhaps one of the hardest parts of the journey. I was so used to being hard on myself, to judging myself harshly for my mistakes. But I realized that if I was going to change, I needed to be gentle with myself. I needed to recognize that change is a process, not a destination, and that it requires patience, perseverance, and a lot of self-love.

In practicing self-compassion, I also learned to set boundaries. I realized that part of being authentic meant honoring my own needs and limits, not just pleasing others or avoiding conflict. I had to learn to say no when I needed to, to protect my time and energy, to prioritize my well-being. Setting boundaries was not easy for me. I had always been a people-pleaser, afraid of rejection or abandonment. But I began to see that setting boundaries was an act of self-respect, a way of honoring myself and my values.

One of the most significant changes I experienced as I built these new habits was a shift in my sense of self-worth. As I let go of manipulation and embraced authenticity, I began to feel more confident, more grounded, more at peace with who I was. I realized that my worth was not dependent on how well I could manipulate others or how much control I had over my environment. My worth was inherent, simply because I was human, because I was alive. This realization was both humbling and empowering.

Building new habits also meant learning to embrace discomfort. Authenticity often meant stepping into the unknown, into the uncertain, into the uncomfortable. It meant being willing to take risks, to face rejection, to be vulnerable. This was scary, but it was also liberating. I began to see that discomfort was not something to be avoided, but something to be embraced, a sign that I was growing, that I was moving forward on my journey toward becoming a more authentic version of myself.

Through this process, I have learned that authenticity is not a destination, but a journey, one that requires constant practice, reflection, and self-awareness. It is not about being perfect or having it all figured out. It is about being real, being honest, being true to oneself. It is about showing up fully, with all our flaws, all our imperfections, and all our humanity. And in doing so, we open ourselves up to deeper connections, more meaningful relationships, and a more fulfilling life.

8.1 Honest Communication: Speaking with Integrity

Communication has always been at the heart of every relationship, whether it's a friendship, a romantic partnership, or a connection with a family member. For most of my life, though, my way of communicating was far from honest. I hid behind a web of words, carefully crafted to manipulate, control, and protect myself. Every conversation was a chess game, every word a move meant to secure an advantage, protect my ego, or avoid vulnerability. This was not communication; it was a constant exercise in self-preservation, a dance designed to keep others at arm's length while maintaining the illusion of connection.

When I embarked on the journey to change, I knew that if I wanted to have meaningful relationships, I needed to unlearn these habits. I needed to learn to communicate with honesty and integrity, to express myself openly without relying on manipulation or deceit. But this was easier said than done. Honest communication is not just about telling the truth. It's about being authentic, being open about my feelings, my needs, my fears, and being willing to hear and accept the truth from others, even when it is uncomfortable or painful. It's about letting go of control and embracing vulnerability.

One of the first lessons I learned in honest communication was that it required me to face my own discomfort with being exposed. For so long, I had hidden behind a mask, afraid of being seen for who I truly was. To communicate honestly, I had to tear down that mask and let people see the real me — flaws, insecurities, fears, and all. I had to admit when I didn't know something, when I was scared, when I had made a mistake. I had to be willing to show up as myself, without pretense or performance. This was terrifying at first. I worried about being judged, rejected, or misunderstood. But I also realized that this fear was the very thing that had been keeping me trapped in old patterns. To break free, I had to confront it head-on.

I started by practicing small acts of honesty in my daily life. At first, it was as simple as admitting when I was wrong, or saying, "I don't know," when I didn't have an answer. I noticed how often I would try to cover up my ignorance or mistakes with excuses or justifications. I caught myself mid-sentence, stopped, and tried again. "I made a mistake," I would say, or "I'm not sure, but I'll find out." This felt awkward, even painful at first, but it also felt refreshing. I was no longer wasting energy trying to appear perfect or all-knowing. I was allowing myself to be human.

I also had to learn to express my needs and desires honestly, without resorting to passive aggression or manipulation. This was one of the hardest parts for me. I had grown accustomed to hinting at what I wanted, making indirect comments, or using guilt to pressure others into giving me what I desired. I believed that if people really cared about me, they would "just know" what I needed. But this was a fantasy. I realized that expecting others to read my mind was not only unfair but also unrealistic. I had to learn to state my needs directly, clearly, and without shame.

The first time I tried this, I remember feeling a surge of anxiety. I was afraid that by expressing my needs openly, I would come across as demanding or selfish. But I pushed through that fear. "I need to feel supported in this decision," I said to a friend, "and it would mean a lot to me if you could be there." To my surprise, my friend responded with understanding and kindness. They were not offended by my honesty; in fact, they appreciated it. This small moment was a revelation. I realized that by communicating my needs openly, I was not pushing people away; I was inviting them to connect with me on a deeper level.

As I continued to practice honest communication, I also had to confront my fear of conflict. I had spent much of my life avoiding difficult conversations, afraid that any disagreement would lead to rejection or abandonment. I would agree to things I didn't want to do, nod along even when I disagreed, and suppress my true feelings to keep the peace. But this avoidance only led to resentment and misunderstandings. I had to learn that conflict was not inherently bad; it was a natural part of any relationship and, when handled with honesty and respect, could actually strengthen connections rather than weaken them.

I started by addressing small conflicts directly and honestly. Instead of bottling up my frustrations, I would speak up when something bothered me. "I feel hurt when you cancel our plans at the last minute," I said to a close friend. "I know things come up, but it makes me feel like I'm not a priority." My voice shook as I spoke, and my heart raced, but I forced myself to stay present, to stay open. To my surprise, my friend responded with empathy and understanding. They apologized, and we were able to talk through the issue in a way that felt healing rather than damaging. I realized then that conflict, when approached with honesty and kindness, could actually bring people closer together.

Learning to communicate honestly also meant embracing empathy — not just for others, but for myself. I had to learn to recognize my own emotions, to sit with them, and to express them in a way that was authentic and compassionate. For years, I had been out of touch with my feelings, numbing myself to avoid pain or discomfort. Now, I had to learn to tune in, to name what I was feeling, and to communicate it openly. "I feel overwhelmed," I would say, or "I'm feeling insecure right now." This was not about blaming others for my feelings, but about owning my emotions and expressing them honestly.

Empathy also meant listening deeply to others. For so long, I had only half-listened in conversations, waiting for my turn to speak, or looking for an opportunity to steer the discussion in a direction that suited me. But honest communication required a different kind of listening — a listening that was full of presence, curiosity, and a genuine desire to understand the other person. I practiced this by asking open-ended questions, by putting aside my assumptions, and by truly tuning into the words, emotions, and needs of the people I was speaking with.

One of the most challenging moments in this journey came when I had to face the truth about my past manipulations. I had to communicate honestly with those I had hurt, to apologize sincerely, and to make amends where I could. This required a level of vulnerability that I had never allowed myself to experience before. I had to be willing to listen to their pain, to accept their anger or disappointment, and to acknowledge the harm I had caused. I had to say, "I hurt you, and I'm sorry," without expecting forgiveness or absolution in return. I had to accept that some wounds take time to heal and that my role was simply to be honest, to listen, and to be present.

In these conversations, I learned that honest communication is not always about saying the right thing; it's about being real. It's about showing up fully, even when it's uncomfortable, even when it's hard. It's about allowing others to see me, not just the polished version I had once tried to present, but the messy, imperfect, and vulnerable human being underneath. It's about creating a space where others feel safe to be real with me in return.

There were times when my honesty was met with resistance or even hostility. Not everyone was ready or willing to engage in the kind of open, honest dialogue I was seeking. I had to learn that this was okay, too. I could not control how others responded to my honesty. I could only control my own actions, my own choices. I had to learn to stay true to my commitment to honest communication, even when it was not reciprocated. I had to learn to let go of my need for approval or validation from others and to trust that, in the long run, honesty would bring the right people into my life and help me build the kind of relationships I truly desired.

As I continued on this path, I discovered that honest communication had another unexpected benefit: it brought me closer to myself. The more I practiced speaking openly and truthfully, the more I began to understand my own needs, desires, and boundaries. I became more in tune with my own emotions, more aware of my own triggers and patterns. I began to see myself with more clarity, more compassion, and more acceptance. I realized that honest communication was not just a tool for connecting with others; it was also a way of connecting with myself.

Over time, I found that honesty became less of a practice and more of a way of being. It became a natural part of how I moved through the world, how I engaged with others, how I expressed myself. I no longer felt the need to manipulate or control; I no longer felt the urge to hide behind a mask or a façade. I felt free to be myself, to speak my truth, to show up fully and authentically in every interaction. This was not about being perfect; it was about being real. It was about embracing the messy, beautiful, imperfect journey of being human.

In this process, I also learned the importance of forgiveness — not just for others, but for myself. I had to forgive myself for the times when I had been dishonest, for the times when I had hurt others, for the times when I had failed to live up to my own values. I had to recognize that change is a journey, not a destination, and that I was bound to stumble along the way. Forgiveness allowed me to let go of guilt and shame and to continue moving forward on my path toward authenticity.

Looking back, I see that learning to communicate honestly has been one of the most transformative aspects of my journey. It has taught me the value of integrity, the power of vulnerability, and the beauty of being true to myself. It has helped me build deeper, more meaningful relationships and has brought a sense of peace and fulfillment that I never thought possible. It has shown me that, in the end, the most important relationship I have is the one with myself. And for that, I am profoundly grateful.

Chapter 9: Self-Forgiveness and Growth – Moving Beyond the Shame

Forgiveness is a word that carries an immense weight, often tied to the idea of letting go of resentment, hurt, or betrayal caused by others. But when the pain is self-inflicted, when the damage comes from one's own actions and choices, forgiveness takes on a different, more challenging meaning. In my journey, the act of self-forgiveness was not merely a moment of grace but a critical turning point—a profound reckoning with the shame that had been festering within me for years. It was the key to my growth, the way forward from the person I had been to the person I longed to become.

For most of my life, I carried a deep, hidden sense of shame, buried beneath layers of denial, anger, and defensiveness. At first, it was just a faint whisper, easily drowned out by the noise of my justifications and excuses. But as I began to confront my narcissistic behaviors and understand the impact they had on others, that whisper grew louder. It evolved into a roar, a relentless inner critic that berated me for my failings, my manipulations, and the pain I had caused. I found myself consumed by regret, unable to escape the constant reminders of what I had done. The more I delved into my past, the more I was confronted with the stark reality of my actions, and the shame felt like an insurmountable wall, blocking any path toward healing or redemption.

I remember the countless nights lying awake, replaying memories of the people I had hurt—the betrayals, the manipulations, the lies. I saw the faces of those who had once trusted me, who had looked to me for love, support, and understanding, and I had failed them. Each memory felt like a stab to the heart, a reminder of how far I had strayed from the person I wanted to be. I was trapped in a vicious cycle: the more I tried to move forward, the more I was dragged back by the weight of my guilt. I knew that to truly change, to truly grow, I had to find a way to forgive myself, but I didn't know where to begin.

Self-forgiveness is not about excusing or minimizing the harm done; it is about acknowledging it fully, taking responsibility, and making a conscious decision to move beyond it. It is an act of courage, a willingness to confront the darkest parts of oneself with compassion rather than condemnation. For me, this process began with accepting the reality of my actions without sugarcoating or rationalizing them. I had to face the hard truth: I had been a narcissist, and I had caused pain. There was no escaping this fact. The only way out was through—to look directly at my shame, my guilt, and my regret, and to sit with it, no matter how uncomfortable it made me feel.

This was perhaps one of the most challenging parts of my journey. My instinct was to run from the pain, to distract myself with anything that could numb the sting of shame. But I soon realized that running would only prolong my suffering. I had to do the opposite; I had to lean in, to allow myself to feel every ounce of the remorse, the sadness, and the regret. I had to be willing to cry, to grieve, to mourn the person I had been, and to acknowledge the hurt I had caused, both to others and to myself. This was not about wallowing in self-pity; it was about honoring the full scope of my experience, about giving space to the feelings I had spent so long avoiding.

In those moments of deep self-reflection, I began to understand that shame, in its most raw form, is a call to action. It is an emotional signal that something needs to change, that there is a misalignment between one's values and one's actions. For so long, I had allowed shame to paralyze me, to keep me stuck in a loop of self-condemnation and despair. But what if I could reframe it? What if, instead of viewing shame as a punishment, I saw it as an opportunity—a chance to grow, to learn, and to become better?

I began to ask myself new questions: What can I learn from this shame? How can I use it to fuel my growth rather than my self-destruction? How can I transform this heavy burden into something lighter, something meaningful? These were not easy questions to answer, but they opened the door to a new way of thinking, one that was grounded in curiosity rather than judgment, in compassion rather than contempt.

One of the most powerful realizations I had was that self-forgiveness is an ongoing process, not a single moment of absolution. It is a practice, something that must be cultivated daily, like a garden that requires constant tending. I started by acknowledging my mistakes openly, both to myself and to those I had hurt. I wrote letters of apology, not with the expectation of forgiveness from others, but as an act of self-expression, a way to release the shame that had been trapped inside me for so long. I apologized not just for my actions, but for the ways in which I had failed to be the person I knew I could be. I acknowledged my humanity, my imperfections, and my deep desire to change.

I also learned to forgive myself for the things I could not control. I had to accept that I was shaped by my past, by my childhood experiences, by my traumas, and by the defenses I had built up to survive. This was not an excuse, but an understanding that I was not inherently "bad" or "evil." I was a person who had made mistakes, who had hurt others, but who was also capable of growth, of change, and of becoming someone better. I had to let go of the idea that I was defined solely by my past, that I was trapped in a narrative of shame and regret. I began to see myself as a work in progress, someone who was learning, evolving, and striving to do better each day.

Self-forgiveness also required me to embrace vulnerability. I had to be willing to open myself up, to share my journey with others, even when it felt uncomfortable or exposing. I had to let go of the fear of judgment and allow myself to be seen for who I truly was—a flawed, imperfect human being, doing the best I could to grow and learn. I started by having honest conversations with those closest to me, sharing my struggles, my regrets, and my desire to make amends. I learned to accept that not everyone would understand or forgive me, and that was okay. My journey was not about seeking validation or approval; it was about finding peace within myself.

One of the most transformative moments came when I realized that self-forgiveness is deeply tied to self-compassion. I had to learn to treat myself with the same kindness and understanding that I would offer to a friend in a similar situation. I had to remind myself that I was worthy of forgiveness, not because I had done anything to earn it, but because I was human, and all humans make mistakes. I practiced self-compassion through daily affirmations, reminding myself that I was enough, that I was capable of change, and that I deserved to be free from the chains of my past.

Growth, I found, comes from this place of compassion. When we forgive ourselves, we create space for new possibilities, for new ways of being in the world. We let go of the need to punish ourselves for past mistakes and instead focus on how we can learn and evolve. I began to set new intentions for myself, to cultivate new habits that aligned with my values. I committed to being more present, more empathetic, and more authentic in my interactions with others. I practiced mindfulness, meditation, and journaling as tools for self-reflection and self-awareness. I made a conscious effort to be kinder to myself, to celebrate my progress, and to be gentle with myself when I stumbled.

The journey of self-forgiveness also taught me the importance of setting boundaries—both with others and with myself. I had to learn to protect my energy, to say no when necessary, and to prioritize my own well-being. I realized that I could not give to others from an empty cup, and that in order to be the person I wanted to be, I needed to take care of myself first. This meant letting go of toxic relationships, setting limits with those who drained me, and being honest about my own needs and limitations. It meant learning to say, "I'm doing the best I can," and believing it.

Moving beyond shame required me to redefine my relationship with myself. I had to shift from seeing myself as someone who was broken, flawed, or beyond redemption, to seeing myself as someone who was whole, capable, and worthy of love and acceptance. I had to learn to trust myself again, to believe in my own capacity for growth and change. This was not an overnight transformation; it was a gradual process, one that required patience, perseverance, and a lot of self-love.

As I continued to practice self-forgiveness, I began to notice a shift in how I viewed the world. I became more compassionate, not just towards myself, but towards others as well. I realized that everyone is fighting their own battles, carrying their own burdens of shame and guilt. I found myself becoming more empathetic, more understanding, and more willing to offer forgiveness to others. I learned that forgiveness, whether of oneself or of others, is not about condoning or excusing harmful behavior; it is about releasing the hold that resentment and anger have on our hearts. It is about choosing love over fear, compassion over judgment, and growth over stagnation.

In embracing self-forgiveness, I found a new sense of freedom—a freedom to be myself, to make mistakes, to learn, and to grow. I discovered that I could be both a work in progress and a masterpiece, that I could hold both my past and my potential in the same breath. I found the courage to let go of the shame that had been weighing me down and to step into a future filled with hope, purpose, and possibility.

Self-forgiveness is not a destination; it is a journey, one that I will continue to walk for the rest of my life. But it is a journey worth taking, for it has led me to a place of peace, of acceptance, and of profound growth. It has allowed me to heal the wounds of my past and to build a future that is rooted in love, compassion, and authenticity. And for that, I am forever grateful.

9.1 Embracing Vulnerability: Allowing Myself to Be Imperfect

There's an immense power in vulnerability—a power I had never truly grasped until I faced the raw and unfiltered truth of my own imperfections. Vulnerability was not a concept I welcomed easily. For years, I had wrapped myself in a thick armor of self-sufficiency, control, and detachment, convincing myself that I was invulnerable, immune to the messy emotions that others seemed so entangled by. I believed that to show vulnerability was to show weakness, and I was determined never to let anyone see me weak. But in truth, my armor was fragile, easily shattered by the slightest touch of fear or doubt.

I was terrified of being imperfect. My entire identity had been built on a foundation of appearing strong, competent, and self-assured. I wore masks that showed the world what I wanted them to see—a persona of invincibility, of having all the answers, of being in control. But beneath those masks lay a deep fear that I was unworthy, that I would never be enough. This fear drove me to manipulate, deceive, and hurt those around me, all in a desperate attempt to hide my perceived flaws.

But hiding my imperfections did not make them disappear. On the contrary, it made them fester in the dark, feeding off my shame and insecurity, growing more powerful and insidious with every attempt to conceal them. It was only when I began to strip away the layers of protection, when I dared to expose the parts of myself that I had long kept hidden, that I began to understand what true strength really was.

Vulnerability is not about baring our souls to anyone and everyone; it's about daring to show up as we are, without the masks, without the pretenses, and without the fear of judgment. It is about being real, honest, and authentic—even when it scares us to the core. It is about owning our story, embracing our imperfections, and recognizing that being human means being flawed. And that is okay.

The first step in embracing vulnerability was admitting to myself that I was afraid—afraid of being rejected, misunderstood, or ridiculed. I had to acknowledge that I had spent so much of my life trying to control how others perceived me, afraid that if they saw the real me, they would walk away. But I realized that the cost of this fear was far too high. In trying to protect myself, I had only isolated myself, cutting myself off from true connection, intimacy, and love.

I remember the moment when I first decided to let my guard down. It was with a close friend, someone who had stood by me through thick and thin, who had seen glimpses of my darkness but had chosen to stay. I sat across from them, my heart pounding in my chest, my palms sweaty with nerves. Every instinct told me to change the subject, to deflect, to make a joke and move on. But something inside me knew that this was a moment of truth.

"I need to tell you something," I began, my voice barely above a whisper. "I've been hiding a lot...about who I am, about what I've done. I've been afraid to show you the real me, because I thought you wouldn't understand, or worse, that you would leave."

I paused, swallowing hard, my throat dry and tight. My friend sat quietly, waiting, their expression gentle, patient. I felt the urge to retreat, to take back my words, but I forced myself to continue.

"I'm not perfect," I confessed, the words feeling foreign and strange in my mouth. "I've made mistakes...many mistakes. I've hurt people, manipulated situations, acted out of fear and insecurity. And I'm not proud of it. But I'm trying to change. I'm trying to be better. And I need you to know that I'm scared...scared of what you'll think of me, scared of being judged, scared of losing you."

My voice cracked on the last word, and I felt the sting of tears in my eyes. I had never felt so exposed, so vulnerable. But instead of the rejection I had feared, my friend reached across the table and took my hand. "Thank you," they said softly. "Thank you for trusting me enough to be honest. We all have our flaws, and it takes courage to own them. I'm here for you, no matter what."

That moment was a revelation. I had allowed myself to be seen, truly seen, in all my messiness and imperfection, and instead of being met with scorn or dismissal, I was met with compassion and acceptance. It was the first time I realized that vulnerability was not a weakness but a strength—a strength that came from the courage to be myself, flaws and all.

From that point on, I began to make a conscious effort to embrace vulnerability in my daily life. It wasn't easy. There were times when I wanted to retreat back into my old habits, to put up walls and pretend that everything was fine. But each time I chose to be open, to share my truth, to let others see the real me, I felt a little bit lighter, a little bit freer. I began to understand that vulnerability was the gateway to connection, to authenticity, to true growth.

Being vulnerable also meant allowing myself to make mistakes and to be okay with that. I had spent so much of my life trying to be perfect, trying to meet an impossible standard that I had set for myself, that I had forgotten what it meant to be human. I had to learn to forgive myself for my imperfections, to accept that I was not always going to get it right, and that that was okay. I had to learn to laugh at my mistakes, to see them not as failures but as opportunities for growth.

One of the most challenging aspects of embracing vulnerability was learning to ask for help. I had always prided myself on being self-reliant, on not needing anyone. But the truth was, I did need others. I needed their support, their guidance, their love. I had to learn to let go of my pride, to admit when I didn't have all the answers, and to reach out to those who could help me on my journey.

I remember the first time I asked for help from my therapist. It felt like a defeat, a sign that I wasn't strong enough to handle things on my own. But as I sat in her office, sharing my fears and insecurities, I realized that asking for help was not a sign of weakness but of strength. It took courage to admit that I needed support, that I couldn't do it all alone. And in doing so, I allowed myself to be held, to be guided, to be loved in a way that I had never experienced before.

Embracing vulnerability also meant learning to be honest with myself about my needs and desires. I had spent so long suppressing my feelings, pretending that I didn't care, that I didn't need or want anything from anyone. But the truth was, I did have needs, I did have desires, and it was okay to acknowledge them. I began to practice self-compassion, to speak to myself with kindness rather than criticism, to honor my own feelings rather than dismissing them.

As I became more comfortable with vulnerability, I noticed a shift in my relationships. I began to attract people who were also willing to be open and honest, who were not afraid to show their own imperfections. I found myself connecting with others on a deeper level, sharing my journey, my struggles, my victories, and learning from theirs. I realized that vulnerability was a gift, not just to myself but to those around me. It created a space for genuine connection, for empathy, for understanding.

I also began to see vulnerability as a form of liberation. By embracing my imperfections, I freed myself from the need to be perfect, from the constant pressure to prove my worth. I began to see myself not as a project that needed fixing but as a whole, complete person who was constantly evolving. I allowed myself to be present in the moment, to experience life fully, without the fear of judgment or rejection. I began to trust that I was enough, just as I was, and that my worth was not tied to my actions or achievements but to my inherent humanity.

There were still moments of doubt, moments when I questioned whether I was doing the right thing, whether I was worthy of love and acceptance. But each time those thoughts crept in, I reminded myself of the power of vulnerability. I reminded myself that it was okay to be imperfect, to have fears, to make mistakes. I reminded myself that vulnerability was not a destination but a journey, one that required patience, courage, and a whole lot of self-love.

And so, I continued to walk this path, embracing my vulnerability, allowing myself to be seen, to be heard, to be known. I learned that being vulnerable was not about being fearless; it was about having the courage to move forward, even in the face of fear. It was about daring to be real, to be honest, to be myself.

By embracing vulnerability, I found a deeper sense of peace, a greater capacity for love, and a renewed sense of purpose. I discovered that my imperfections were not something to be ashamed of but something to be celebrated. They were a testament to my growth, to my resilience, to my journey toward becoming my truest self.

In allowing myself to be imperfect, I gave myself the freedom to be human, to live fully, to love deeply, and to embrace the beautiful, messy, complex experience that is life. And in doing so, I found a strength I never knew I had—a strength that came not from hiding my vulnerabilities but from owning them, from letting them shine, from letting them guide me on the path to true healing and transformation.

Part 3: Thriving After Narcissism - Practical Tools and New Perspectives

Chapter 10: Tools for Ongoing Change – Daily Practices and Mindfulness

Change isn't a destination; it's a continuous journey, a daily commitment to becoming a better version of ourselves. For me, embracing change meant not only transforming my mindset but also creating routines and practices that would support this new way of living. I had spent years living in a state of denial and avoidance, afraid to confront my true self, but I knew that lasting change required me to face my flaws head-on. It required me to commit to new habits, to mindfulness, to a life of intentional growth.

In the early days of my transformation, I believed that change was about grand gestures, about making sweeping promises to myself and others. I thought that if I could just do one big thing—say the right words, offer the perfect apology, take some bold action—it would magically erase the past and reset my future. But as the days turned into weeks, I realized that true change wasn't about the grand gestures at all. It was about the small, seemingly insignificant choices I made every single day.

Daily practices and mindfulness became the foundation of my journey toward lasting change. I had to learn to be present, to be aware of my thoughts, my emotions, and my actions. I had to learn to interrupt the automatic patterns of behavior that had governed my life for so long. It wasn't easy; in fact, it was one of the hardest things I had ever done. But I soon discovered that the smallest steps, when taken consistently, had the power to create the most profound transformation.

One of the first practices I incorporated into my daily routine was mindfulness meditation. I had heard about meditation for years but had always dismissed it as something too "woo-woo" or new-agey for me. I couldn't imagine sitting still with my thoughts, especially when my mind felt like a stormy sea, churning with self-doubt, shame, and regret. But I also knew that if I wanted to change, I had to be willing to try something new.

At first, meditation felt like torture. Sitting still, focusing on my breath, trying to quiet my mind—it was all too much. My thoughts raced, my body fidgeted, and I felt like I was doing it all wrong. But instead of giving up, I chose to stay with the discomfort. I learned to observe my thoughts without judgment, to notice when my mind wandered and gently bring it back to my breath. I learned to breathe deeply, to ground myself in the present moment, and to accept whatever arose, without resistance.

Over time, meditation became less of a struggle and more of a refuge. I began to notice subtle shifts in my thinking. I became more aware of my triggers, more attuned to my emotions. I realized that I didn't have to be a slave to my thoughts—that I could choose which thoughts to entertain and which to let go. Meditation helped me cultivate a sense of inner peace, a calmness that allowed me to approach each day with more clarity and intention.

In addition to meditation, I started practicing gratitude. This might sound cliché, but expressing gratitude was a game-changer for me. For so long, I had focused on what was wrong with my life—what I didn't have, what I had lost, what I had failed to achieve. My mind was constantly scanning for the negative, always on high alert for any sign of threat or disappointment. Gratitude helped me shift my focus, to see the beauty and blessings that were already present in my life.

Each morning, I began a practice of writing down three things I was grateful for. At first, it felt forced and awkward. I struggled to find anything worth mentioning, and the exercise felt like a hollow ritual. But I persisted. I wrote down even the smallest things—a warm cup of coffee, the sound of birds outside my window, a kind word from a stranger. And slowly, I began to notice a change. I began to feel a sense of abundance, a deep appreciation for the simple moments that made up my day. Gratitude became a lens through which I could view the world, a tool that helped me see beyond my fears and insecurities.

Mindfulness wasn't just about meditation and gratitude, though. It was about being fully present in every aspect of my life. It was about noticing the way I spoke to others, the way I treated myself, the way I reacted to challenges. I started paying attention to the words I used, both in my internal dialogue and in my conversations with others. I realized that I often spoke harshly, that I used language that was self-defeating or judgmental. I made a conscious effort to choose my words more carefully, to speak with kindness and compassion, not just to others but to myself.

One of the most transformative practices I adopted was mindful breathing. Whenever I felt overwhelmed or anxious, I would take a few deep breaths, inhaling slowly through my nose, holding the breath for a few moments, and then exhaling through my mouth. It sounds so simple, but it had an immediate calming effect. It helped me pause, to step back from whatever situation was triggering me, and to respond with intention rather than react out of habit. Mindful breathing became a way for me to ground myself, to return to the present moment, and to remind myself that I had the power to choose my response.

Another daily practice that supported my journey was journaling. I had always been a bit skeptical about journaling, thinking it was something people did in their teenage years, not in adulthood. But I quickly realized the power of putting my thoughts down on paper. Journaling allowed me to process my emotions, to reflect on my experiences, and to gain insights that I might not have otherwise discovered. It became a safe space where I could be honest with myself, where I could explore my fears, my hopes, my dreams, without judgment.

Through journaling, I began to see patterns in my behavior. I noticed how often I defaulted to defensiveness, how I would shut down when I felt threatened, how I would avoid uncomfortable conversations rather than confront them. But I also began to see my progress, to recognize the small victories along the way—the times when I chose to be honest, when I allowed myself to be vulnerable, when I made the choice to be kind rather than defensive. Journaling became a mirror that reflected my growth, that showed me how far I had come and where I still needed to go.

Alongside these practices, I embraced the concept of self-care. For years, I had viewed self-care as selfish or indulgent, something that only people with too much time on their hands bothered with. But I soon realized that self-care was essential to my healing. It wasn't about bubble baths or spa days; it was about honoring my needs, setting boundaries, and taking care of my mental, emotional, and physical well-being. I learned to listen to my body, to recognize when I needed rest, when I needed nourishment, when I needed to step back and recharge.

I began to create a daily routine that included exercise, healthy eating, and plenty of sleep. I discovered the joy of moving my body, whether it was through yoga, walking, or dancing. I found that physical activity not only helped me stay healthy but also lifted my mood, reduced anxiety, and boosted my confidence. I made a commitment to nourish my body with whole, healthy foods, recognizing that what I put into my body had a direct impact on my energy, my mood, and my overall well-being. And I made sleep a priority, understanding that rest was not a luxury but a necessity for my body and mind to heal.

Mindfulness also meant learning to say no, to set boundaries, to protect my energy. I had spent so much of my life trying to please others, trying to be everything to everyone, that I had forgotten how to take care of myself. I had to learn that it was okay to say no, that it was okay to prioritize my needs, that it was okay to walk away from situations or people that drained me. Setting boundaries was not easy; it required me to confront my fears of rejection, my need for approval, my discomfort with conflict. But it also empowered me, giving me a sense of control over my life and my choices.

Daily practices and mindfulness became my anchors, the tools that grounded me in my commitment to change. They helped me stay present, to be aware of my thoughts, to choose my actions with intention. They reminded me that change wasn't something that happened overnight, that it wasn't a destination to be reached but a journey to be embraced. And as I continued to practice these tools, day in and day out, I began to see the fruits of my labor. I began to feel more at peace, more connected, more alive. I began to trust myself, to believe in my ability to change, to know that I was capable of becoming the person I wanted to be.

But perhaps most importantly, I began to understand that the journey of change is never really over. It is a daily commitment, a choice we make every single day to show up, to be present, to be honest, to be kind, to be our truest selves. And as I continue on this path, I know that I will stumble, I will fall, I will make mistakes. But I also know that I have the tools, the practices, the mindfulness to pick myself up, to keep going, to keep growing.

Change is not a one-time event; it is a lifetime journey. It is about becoming the person we are meant to be, not by erasing our past but by learning from it, by embracing our imperfections, by choosing every day to live with intention, with mindfulness, with love. And as I walk this path, I know that I am not alone. I know that there are others on this journey with me, others who are also choosing to change, to grow, to become their best selves. And together, we can support each other, encourage each other, and remind each other that we are all capable of change, that we are all capable of becoming who we are meant to be.

10.1 Morning Rituals: Setting a Positive Tone for the Day

When I began this journey of transformation, I underestimated the power of mornings. For years, my mornings were filled with anxiety, irritation, and a feeling of dread. I would wake up and immediately reach for my phone, scrolling through emails or social media, allowing external forces to set the tone for my day. It felt like I was always running against the clock, overwhelmed by the demands of the day before it even began. I didn't realize that I was giving away the first and most precious moments of each day to chaos, fear, and negativity.

As I started to take responsibility for my behavior and work on becoming a better person, I realized that how I began each day had a massive impact on how I lived it. My therapist once told me, "Mornings are like the foundation of a house. If the foundation is shaky, the whole house will eventually crumble." That simple statement changed everything for me. I decided to build a solid foundation for my days, and I started by focusing on my morning rituals.

Creating new morning habits wasn't easy, especially given my natural inclination to fall back into old patterns of control and manipulation. Yet, I realized that if I could take charge of my mornings, I could set a positive tone for my entire day. I wanted to start the day with intention, with a sense of purpose and clarity, rather than letting it unravel into a series of reactive responses to whatever came my way.

The first thing I did was decide to get up earlier, giving myself time to breathe and think before diving into the responsibilities and distractions of life. Instead of hitting the snooze button repeatedly, I made a commitment to rise at a specific time, regardless of how I felt. This simple act of discipline helped me build trust with myself — a trust that had been deeply eroded by years of narcissistic tendencies and self-sabotage.

I also decided to create a ritual of gratitude as soon as I woke up. Gratitude did not come naturally to me at first. In my old mindset, I was far too focused on what I didn't have or what wasn't going right. But I learned that by starting each morning with three things I was grateful for, no matter how small or seemingly insignificant, I could shift my perspective. The first morning, it felt awkward; I struggled to find things I truly appreciated. But over time, it became a grounding force in my life. I began to notice the small joys — the sound of birds outside my window, the warmth of my bed, the simple fact that I had another day to try again. Gratitude started to change me from the inside out.

Mindfulness was another essential aspect of my morning routine. Instead of rushing through my day, I began my mornings with a few minutes of mindful breathing. I would sit quietly, breathe deeply, and focus on the sensation of the air filling my lungs. At first, my mind would race, and it felt almost impossible to sit still. But with practice, I learned to observe my thoughts without getting caught up in them. This practice taught me to be more present, less reactive, and more open to experiencing each moment as it came.

I found that movement, even gentle movement, was vital for me to start my day with energy and focus. I would stretch, do a few yoga poses, or take a brisk walk outside. Moving my body first thing in the morning helped me to release tension and anxiety. It also allowed me to connect with myself physically, reminding me that I was here, alive, and capable of making positive choices.

Another crucial element of my morning ritual was affirmations. Affirmations felt uncomfortable at first. I would stand in front of the mirror, feeling ridiculous as I told myself things like, "I am worthy of love and respect," or "I am committed to my growth and healing." It felt like a lie. But as the days went on, I realized these words were not declarations of where I was at that moment, but affirmations of where I wanted to go. They were seeds I was planting, hoping that in time they would grow into something real. And they did. Slowly but surely, I began to believe those words, and more importantly, I began to act in ways that reflected them.

I also learned to set intentions for the day. Instead of allowing the day to dictate my mood or actions, I would decide how I wanted to show up. I would ask myself questions like, "How do I want to feel today?" or "What kind of energy do I want to bring to my interactions?" Setting these intentions made me more conscious of my behavior and choices throughout the day. If I found myself slipping back into old patterns of defensiveness or manipulation, I could pause, remember my intention, and choose a different path.

One of the hardest but most transformative parts of my morning routine was choosing to stay away from my phone and other digital distractions for at least the first hour of the day. This boundary was a game-changer. It allowed me to reclaim my mornings, to focus on my thoughts and emotions without the noise of the outside world crashing in. I realized how much of my anxiety had been driven by the constant influx of information and the feeling that I always had to be "on" or connected. Disconnecting for even a short while helped me reconnect with myself.

I also began incorporating a brief time of reflection and journaling into my mornings. Journaling became a sacred space for me to pour out my thoughts, fears, dreams, and everything in between. It became a tool for self-discovery and healing. I used it to track my progress, to acknowledge my setbacks without judgment, and to remind myself of the commitment I had made to change. This practice was both grounding and liberating, giving me a way to externalize my internal journey.

As these rituals became habits, I noticed profound changes in my life. I felt more centered, more at peace, and more in control of my emotions. I began to see mornings as a gift, a time to nourish my soul before the world demanded my attention. It was as if I had found a hidden treasure, a source of strength that had been there all along, waiting for me to discover it.

These morning rituals were not just about starting the day positively; they were about reclaiming my power, about deciding that I was worth the time and effort it took to set my day on the right path. They were about acknowledging my past without being defined by it and believing in the possibility of a future filled with authenticity and connection.

There were days, of course, when I slipped, when I reverted to old habits or let the demands of the day take over. But instead of falling into the trap of self-criticism, I chose to see these moments as opportunities for growth. Each morning was a new chance to try again, to choose differently, to reinforce the habits that were slowly but surely changing my life.

Morning rituals became a reflection of the person I was becoming — someone who could face the day with clarity and courage, someone who was learning to let go of the need to control and instead embrace the beauty of each new day.

Chapter 11: Reinventing Relationships – Building Trust from Scratch

There was a time when relationships felt like battlegrounds. I saw every interaction as a challenge, every connection as a way to validate my worth, and every person as someone who either fed my ego or threatened it. Trust wasn't something I believed in; it was something I manipulated, withheld, or weaponized. If I'm honest, my relationships were built on a fragile foundation of control, fear, and dominance. And when things went wrong, as they often did, I was left standing amidst the rubble, wondering why everyone seemed to walk away or keep me at arm's length.

Rebuilding trust—real, authentic trust—was one of the most challenging parts of my journey. I had to acknowledge that I had deeply hurt those who tried to care for me, those who believed in me, and those who saw through my facade yet stayed anyway, hoping for a glimpse of the person they believed I could be. I had broken promises, played emotional games, and pushed people away, all while blaming them for not understanding me or meeting my needs. Now, it was time to face the reality of what I had done and understand how to start again.

Trust, I learned, is not given; it is earned. And earning trust, especially after breaking it, requires more than just an apology or an acknowledgment of past wrongs. It requires consistency, patience, humility, and a willingness to change. It demands actions that align with words, time and time again, until the people around you begin to believe that maybe, just maybe, you are different from who you once were.

I had to start from scratch, with no expectations that anyone owed me their trust or forgiveness. I began with small steps, understanding that trust is not a destination but a journey, a series of moments where you choose to show up differently than you have before. I needed to understand that trust was fragile, like glass that, once shattered, might never be restored to its original form but could still be pieced back together, though with visible cracks and imperfections.

The first step was acknowledging my past behavior without justification or excuses. I needed to be honest about the ways I had manipulated others, the lies I had told, and the damage I had caused. It was humbling, even humiliating, to admit these things, not just to others but to myself. I had to strip away the layers of defensiveness, of self-justification, and face the stark truth of my actions. I realized that if I wanted others to trust me, I had to show that I was willing to trust them first—with my vulnerability, my flaws, and my commitment to change.

Next came the process of asking for forgiveness—not in a way that demanded it, but as an offering of sincerity and a willingness to make amends. I understood that forgiveness, like trust, is not something you are entitled to; it is something you must earn. I reached out to those I had hurt, not to beg for their forgiveness but to take responsibility for my actions, to listen to their pain without defense, and to ask what I could do to make things right. Some were willing to engage, while others were not. I had to learn to accept both responses with grace.

In these early stages, I realized that rebuilding trust also meant learning to trust myself. I had to develop a sense of self-trust by becoming more self-aware and acknowledging the thoughts and impulses that had led me down the wrong path in the past. I started to see that if I didn't trust my own ability to act with integrity, how could I expect others to trust me? This realization prompted a deeper level of self-reflection and commitment to my own growth.

Building new relationships, and mending old ones, required me to approach every interaction with a fresh perspective. I could no longer see others as pawns in my game, but as individuals with their own stories, their own pain, and their own worth. This meant practicing empathy in every conversation, listening more than I spoke, and seeking to understand rather than be understood. It required me to drop my defenses, to stop trying to prove myself, and instead, to just be myself, flaws and all.

One of the most challenging aspects of this process was dealing with the fear that people would never see me as anything but my past mistakes. There were moments when I wanted to give up, to retreat back into old patterns where I felt safer, more in control. But I had to remind myself that trust was not about immediate results but about consistent, authentic effort over time. It was about being willing to sit in the discomfort of being seen for who I really was, without masks or pretenses, and letting others decide for themselves if they wanted to continue the journey with me.

In building new relationships, I made a conscious choice to surround myself with people who embodied the qualities I aspired to—honesty, kindness, compassion, and integrity. I sought out mentors, friends, and even professional guides who could model what healthy, trusting relationships looked like. I paid attention to how they navigated conflicts, how they communicated, and how they showed up for themselves and others. Slowly, I began to understand that trust is not just about grand gestures or declarations; it is built in the small, everyday moments when you choose to show up with honesty, even when it's hard, especially when it's hard.

A significant part of rebuilding trust was learning to apologize, not just with words but with actions. I learned that saying "I'm sorry" means little if it is not followed by a change in behavior. I had to show, through my actions, that I was committed to doing better, to being better. This meant being reliable—if I said I would do something, I did it. If I promised to show up, I showed up. It meant being honest, even when honesty was uncomfortable or when it put me in a vulnerable position.

I also had to practice forgiveness—not just asking for it, but giving it. I realized that holding onto grudges, even against myself, was a form of control, a way to keep my walls up and protect myself from feeling too deeply. But forgiveness, I learned, was an act of release. It was about letting go of the need to be right, the need to win, and instead choosing to be free.

One of the most transformative lessons I learned was that trust is built in the mundane, not the monumental. It is built in showing up every day, being present, being honest, and being kind. It is built in the way you listen, the way you speak, the way you handle disappointment, and the way you celebrate others. It is built in the spaces between words, in the silences that allow for reflection and understanding.

Reinventing relationships was not just about rebuilding trust with others; it was about building a new relationship with myself. It was about learning to trust my instincts, to honor my feelings, and to believe in my capacity to change. It was about letting go of the narrative that I was broken or unworthy and embracing the idea that I was capable of growth and transformation.

There were setbacks along the way, moments when I fell back into old patterns of defensiveness or fear. But I learned that trust is not about perfection; it is about persistence. It is about recognizing when you have strayed off course, acknowledging it, and finding your way back. It is about being gentle with yourself while holding yourself accountable, about finding balance between self-compassion and self-discipline.

As I continued on this journey, I found that trust became less about what others thought of me and more about how I felt about myself. I began to trust myself more—to trust my capacity for growth, for empathy, for love. And as I built that trust within, it started to radiate outward, drawing in people who were willing to walk this path with me, who were willing to give me a chance to show up differently than I had before.

Reinventing relationships became less about proving myself and more about simply being myself, in all my imperfect, messy humanity. It was about understanding that trust is not a fixed state, but a dynamic process—a dance between two people who are willing to be open, vulnerable, and real with each other.

The process of building trust from scratch was humbling, sometimes painful, but ultimately, it was liberating. It taught me that while I could not change the past, I could choose to live differently in the present. I could choose to be someone who builds up rather than tears down, who loves rather than controls, who trusts rather than fears. And in that choice, I found a freedom I had never known—a freedom to be fully, authentically myself and to connect with others in a way that was real, meaningful, and true.

11.1 Creating New Connections: Building Friendships with Authenticity

Rebuilding connections from the ground up was perhaps one of the hardest things I ever set out to do. For years, I had approached relationships with a hidden agenda, consciously or unconsciously evaluating everyone I met on the basis of what they could offer me—admiration, validation, power, or some other form of ego sustenance. I had learned to see people as pawns in a game, characters in a script where I always needed to play the leading role. Friendships were transactions; every word spoken, every gesture made, every action taken was geared towards fulfilling my own needs.

But somewhere along the way, I began to feel the emptiness of it all. The friendships I thought I had built turned out to be as fragile as a house of cards. They crumbled at the first sign of conflict, disagreement, or challenge. I found myself surrounded by people, yet feeling profoundly alone. It became clear that in order to truly create new connections, I needed to approach friendships from a completely different perspective—a perspective rooted not in self-interest, but in authenticity.

Authenticity, I realized, was something I had always struggled with. I had spent so much of my life wearing masks, playing roles, and presenting a version of myself that I thought others would find appealing, acceptable, or admirable. But this was not who I truly was, and deep down, I knew it. To build real friendships, I had to start by dropping the masks and allowing my true self to be seen, flaws and all.

This journey began with a deep dive into self-awareness. I had to confront some hard truths about the ways I had interacted with others. I had to ask myself, "Who am I, really? What do I value? What kind of people do I genuinely want in my life?" I had to face the uncomfortable fact that my previous relationships had often been based on superficial qualities—shared interests, mutual benefits, or even just proximity—rather than on shared values or genuine connections.

The first step in creating new connections was learning to approach people with honesty and vulnerability. This was terrifying at first. Vulnerability had always felt like a weakness, a risk I couldn't afford to take. But as I slowly began to open up, I realized that vulnerability was not a weakness at all; it was a strength. It allowed me to be seen for who I really was, and in doing so, it created a space for others to do the same.

I started small, reaching out to people in my life who had always been there in the background—acquaintances I had never truly engaged with, people I had dismissed because they didn't seem "useful" to me. I began initiating conversations without any ulterior motives, simply to get to know them better. I listened more than I spoke, and when I did speak, I made a conscious effort to share my genuine thoughts and feelings rather than what I thought they wanted to hear.

To my surprise, many of these interactions blossomed into meaningful friendships. I realized that people respond positively to authenticity. When they feel that you are genuinely interested in them—not for what they can do for you, but for who they are—they open up in return. They begin to trust you, and a foundation for a real connection is laid.

As I continued on this path, I learned that creating new connections also required a certain level of discernment. I had to be mindful of whom I allowed into my life. Not everyone was going to be a healthy or positive influence. I needed to learn to recognize the difference between relationships that were nurturing and supportive and those that were toxic or draining. This meant setting boundaries—not as a means of control, but as a way of protecting my newfound authenticity and peace.

Boundaries were something I had struggled with for most of my life. I had always seen them as walls, barriers that kept people out. But I began to understand that boundaries were not walls; they were filters. They allowed me to let the right people in while keeping out those who didn't align with my values or who posed a threat to my emotional well-being.

One of the most important lessons I learned in this process was the importance of mutual respect. I realized that for a friendship to be authentic, it must be based on a foundation of respect. Respect for each other's boundaries, respect for each other's feelings, and respect for each other's individuality. In the past, I had often tried to mold people to fit my own needs or expectations, but I began to understand that true friendship is about acceptance, not control. It's about appreciating people for who they are, not who you want them to be.

Building friendships with authenticity also meant learning to be present. I had to learn to show up fully in my interactions, to be genuinely engaged and attentive rather than distracted or preoccupied with my own thoughts and agendas. This required me to practice mindfulness, to be aware of my own thoughts and feelings in each moment, and to let go of the need to control the outcome of every conversation.

I began to see that being present also meant being patient. Friendships do not develop overnight. They require time, effort, and a willingness to weather the ups and downs that inevitably come with getting to know someone on a deeper level. I had to learn to be okay with the uncomfortable silences, the misunderstandings, and the moments of tension. I had to learn that these moments were not signs of failure, but opportunities for growth and deeper understanding.

As I practiced these principles, I noticed a profound change in the quality of my relationships. The connections I began to form were deeper, more meaningful, and more fulfilling than anything I had experienced before. I found myself surrounded by people who genuinely cared for me, who challenged me to be better, and who accepted me for who I was. I no longer felt the need to prove myself or to play games to keep people in my life. I could simply be myself, and that was enough.

I also learned the importance of gratitude in building authentic friendships. I made a conscious effort to express my appreciation for the people in my life, to acknowledge their kindness, their support, and their presence. I realized that gratitude was a powerful way to strengthen connections, to make people feel valued and seen. It was also a way to keep myself grounded, to remind myself of the beauty and richness of the connections I was creating.

Another key aspect of building friendships with authenticity was learning to be forgiving—both of myself and of others. I had to accept that I was not always going to get it right, that I would make mistakes, and that so would the people I cared about. I had to learn to let go of grudges, to move past disagreements, and to focus on the bigger picture. I realized that holding onto resentment only created barriers to connection, while forgiveness opened the door to deeper understanding and growth.

There were moments when I doubted myself when I wondered if I was truly capable of building genuine connections. There were times when I felt vulnerable and exposed when I questioned whether people would accept me for who I was. But each time I pushed through those fears, each time I chose to be authentic rather than retreat behind a mask, I found that the rewards far outweighed the risks.

In creating new connections, I learned that authenticity is not about being perfect; it's about being real. It's about showing up as you are, in all your messiness and complexity, and allowing others to do the same. It's about finding the courage to be vulnerable, the strength to be honest, and the wisdom to be discerning.

Looking back, I can see that this journey of building friendships with authenticity has not only transformed my relationships with others, but it has also transformed my relationship with myself. I have learned to trust myself more, to believe in my capacity for growth and change, and to embrace the messiness of being human. I have learned that it is okay to be imperfect, to make mistakes, and to learn from them.

Most importantly, I have learned that true connection is not something you find; it is something you create. It is built moment by moment, through every word, every action, and every choice you make to show up with honesty, kindness, and authenticity. And in that creation, I have found a sense of belonging, a sense of peace, and a sense of purpose that I never knew was possible.

11.2 Navigating Family Dynamics: Establishing Healthy Boundaries

Family is a complex landscape, full of history, shared memories, and deep-rooted emotions. For much of my life, I viewed my family through the lens of what they could do for me—how they could validate my worth, reinforce my image, or support my desires. I expected them to conform to my needs and beliefs, and when they didn't, I would react with manipulation, criticism, or silent disdain. I saw myself as the protagonist in a story where everyone else was just a supporting character, playing their parts to fit the narrative I had created.

It wasn't until I began my journey out of narcissism that I realized how deeply flawed this perspective was and how much damage it had caused. My family dynamics were fraught with tension and misunderstandings. Conversations often felt like battles, with each of us fighting to be heard, seen, and understood but rarely achieving any of those things. I felt misunderstood, unappreciated, and unloved, often unaware that my own behavior was the root of many of these conflicts.

To truly heal and transform these dynamics, I needed to learn the art of establishing healthy boundaries—something I had never been good at. I had always seen boundaries as a way to control others or to assert dominance. But I came to understand that boundaries are not about pushing people away; they are about protecting yourself and the relationships that matter to you. They are about creating space for mutual respect, understanding, and healthy interaction.

The first step in establishing boundaries with my family was to recognize the patterns of behavior that were causing harm. I had to identify the ways I would overstep others' boundaries or allow mine to be violated. I realized that I had a tendency to react defensively to any perceived criticism or slight, often escalating situations that could have been resolved with calm, honest communication. I also recognized that I had been using guilt and emotional manipulation to get my way, whether it was seeking sympathy, imposing my opinions, or expecting others to cater to my needs.

Confronting these patterns was uncomfortable and, at times, painful. It required a great deal of self-reflection and a willingness to see myself through the eyes of those I loved. I had to accept that my behavior had often been hurtful and unfair and that I needed to change if I wanted healthier, more fulfilling relationships with my family.

One of the most significant realizations I had was that healthy boundaries start with self-awareness. I had to be clear about what I needed and what I was willing to accept. I had to understand my own triggers and vulnerabilities, as well as those of my family members. This required me to develop empathy—not just for myself, but for them as well. I had to see them as whole, complex individuals with their own needs, fears, and desires, rather than simply as extensions of myself or obstacles to my happiness.

Once I had this understanding, I began to practice setting clear and respectful boundaries. I started small, with straightforward situations where I felt safe to express my needs. For example, I began by letting my family know when I needed time to myself or when a conversation topic was too sensitive or triggering for me. I learned to use "I" statements, such as "I feel overwhelmed when we discuss this," rather than blaming or accusing them with "you" statements. This shift in language made a world of difference. It communicated that I was taking ownership of my feelings and needs, rather than projecting them onto others.

At first, there was resistance. My family wasn't used to this new version of me—one that didn't resort to manipulation or guilt to get my way, but instead spoke honestly and openly about my needs. There were moments when they pushed back, confused by my change in behavior or uncertain how to respond. But slowly, they began to see that my intention wasn't to control them or distance myself, but to create a healthier dynamic that allowed us all to feel safe and respected.

I learned that establishing boundaries is not a one-time event, but an ongoing process. It required constant communication, patience, and a willingness to stand firm in my convictions, even when it felt uncomfortable. There were times when I had to remind myself why I was doing this, especially when faced with resistance or misunderstanding. I had to trust that by honoring my own needs and respecting those of others, I was paving the way for deeper, more meaningful connections.

One of the most challenging aspects of setting boundaries was dealing with the guilt and fear that often came with it. I had to confront the worry that my family might see me as selfish or unloving, or that they might feel hurt or rejected by my new approach. I had to remind myself that setting boundaries wasn't about being unkind or dismissive; it was about being honest and caring enough to show up authentically, without resentment or hidden agendas.

I also had to accept that not everyone would react positively to my boundaries. Some family members found it difficult to adjust to the new dynamics, especially those who were accustomed to a more enmeshed or codependent relationship. I had to come to terms with the fact that I couldn't control their reactions, and that their discomfort was not a reflection of my worth or the validity of my needs.

Through this process, I discovered that setting boundaries also meant learning to say no without feeling guilty or obligated to explain myself. This was incredibly freeing. I realized that I didn't always have to justify my decisions or seek approval for my choices. I could simply honor my own needs and trust that those who truly cared for me would respect my right to do so.

I began to see that boundaries are a way of showing respect—for myself and for others. They are not about keeping people out, but about creating a space where both parties can thrive, free from manipulation, guilt, or resentment. I found that when I approached boundaries with compassion and clarity, rather than defensiveness or fear, they became tools for growth and healing rather than weapons of control.

A pivotal moment in my journey was when I realized that boundaries also apply to how we communicate and engage with our family members. I began to practice active listening, making a conscious effort to really hear what my family was saying, rather than jumping to conclusions or interrupting with my own opinions. I learned to ask questions instead of making assumptions and to validate their feelings even when I didn't agree with their perspectives. This shift in communication opened the door to deeper understanding and empathy, and helped to dissolve the tension that had often plagued our interactions.

There were still moments of conflict, misunderstandings, and hurt feelings. But instead of avoiding these moments or responding with anger, I began to see them as opportunities for growth. I started to view each conflict as a chance to practice the skills I was learning—to communicate more effectively, to stand firm in my boundaries, and to approach each situation with empathy and understanding.

One of the hardest boundaries I had to set was with myself. I had to learn to let go of the need for approval, to accept that not everyone in my family would agree with or understand my choices. I had to remind myself that my worth was not dependent on their validation, and that it was okay to disappoint people if it meant staying true to myself.

I also had to learn to forgive myself for past mistakes. I had to accept that I was not perfect, that I had caused harm, and that all I could do now was strive to be better. I realized that forgiveness was a form of self-compassion, a way of acknowledging my humanity and allowing myself to move forward without the weight of shame or regret.

Over time, I noticed a profound change in my family dynamics. Conversations became more open and honest, less charged with hidden agendas or unspoken resentments. I felt more at peace in my interactions, more confident in my ability to communicate my needs, and more accepting of others' boundaries. I found that my family members began to mirror this behavior, setting their own boundaries and respecting mine in turn.

Navigating family dynamics and establishing healthy boundaries is not an easy task. It requires patience, persistence, and a willingness to face discomfort and uncertainty. But it is also incredibly rewarding. It has allowed me to create deeper, more authentic connections with the people I love, and to feel more grounded and secure in myself.

I have come to see that boundaries are not about building walls, but about creating bridges—bridges that connect us to others in a way that is honest, respectful, and sustainable. They are tools that help us navigate the complexities of family life, allowing us to love more fully and freely, without losing ourselves in the process.

Chapter 12: From Self-Centered to Self-Aware – Creating a Purposeful Life

For the longest time, I believed that life's purpose revolved around my needs, desires, and ambitions. I was convinced that my happiness was something to be pursued with relentless intensity, as though it existed in some far-off destination, a place I could reach if only I pushed hard enough, demanded enough, or took enough from the world around me. I saw myself as the center of every story, the sun around which everything else revolved. And for a while, this perspective seemed to work. It gave me a sense of control, of being powerful in a world that felt chaotic and unpredictable.

But deep down, I felt an emptiness that gnawed at me. It was a void that no amount of validation, success, or admiration could fill. I was constantly striving for more—more recognition, more praise, more of the things I believed would finally make me feel whole. But the more I sought, the more hollow I felt. It was as though I was pouring water into a cup with no bottom. Nothing ever seemed to be enough.

Then, as I began my journey out of narcissism, I started to realize that the problem wasn't that I needed more; it was that I needed something entirely different. I needed purpose—not the kind of purpose that revolves around self-aggrandizement or external validation, but a deeper, more meaningful purpose that connected me to something beyond myself. I needed to learn how to shift from being self-centered to becoming truly self-aware.

Self-awareness, I discovered, is not just about knowing your strengths or weaknesses, your likes or dislikes. It's about understanding who you are at your core, what you value, and how you want to show up in the world. It's about recognizing your impact on others and taking responsibility for the energy you bring into every room you enter. It's about looking beyond the surface and diving into the depths of your own mind and soul to uncover the person you are meant to become.

The first step in this process was letting go of the need for constant approval and validation. For years, I had built my sense of self on what others thought of me—on the compliments, the admiration, the affirmation. But I began to see that this was a fragile foundation, one that could crumble at any moment. I realized that if I wanted to build a meaningful life, I had to learn to validate myself, to find my worth within, rather than in the eyes of others.

This was not an easy task. It meant facing the parts of myself I had long ignored—the parts that were insecure, afraid, or uncertain. It meant confronting my own shadows, my doubts, and my fears. But as I did this work, I began to notice a shift. I started to feel a quiet confidence, a sense of inner peace that I had never known before. I realized that my worth was not something that could be given or taken away by anyone else. It was something that was intrinsic to who I was.

As I grew in self-awareness, I began to explore what truly mattered to me—what I was passionate about, what brought me joy, what made me feel alive. I started asking myself questions I had never dared to ask before: What kind of life do I want to create? What values do I want to live by? What legacy do I want to leave behind? These questions became the guiding compass for my journey towards a more purposeful life.

One of the most important realizations I had was that purpose is not something you find; it's something you create. It's not a destination you arrive at one day, but a path you choose to walk every single day. It's about making conscious choices that align with your values and priorities, about being intentional in your actions and decisions. I realized that I didn't have to wait for some grand epiphany or life-changing event to start living with purpose; I could start right where I was, with the small, everyday choices I made.

I began to identify the things that genuinely mattered to me—the causes I cared about, the passions I wanted to pursue, the impact I wanted to have on the people around me. I realized that my purpose was not about impressing others or achieving some external standard of success, but about living in a way that felt true and authentic to me. It was about finding fulfillment in the journey itself, rather than in any specific outcome.

One of the biggest shifts I made was in my relationships. I started to see them not as vehicles for my own validation or satisfaction, but as opportunities to connect, to give, and to grow. I began to approach my interactions with others with a sense of curiosity and openness, rather than a desire to control or manipulate. I learned to listen more deeply, to seek to understand rather than to be understood. I discovered that there is a profound joy in being truly present with someone, in witnessing their journey and sharing in their experiences, without needing to make it about myself.

I also found that purpose often comes from service— from giving of yourself in a way that uplifts, inspires, or supports others. I began to explore ways I could use my own experiences, my own story, to help others on their journeys. I started volunteering, mentoring, and sharing my insights with those who were struggling with similar challenges. I found that in giving of myself, I was also receiving something far more valuable than I had ever imagined. I was finding a sense of connection, of community, and of meaning that went far beyond anything I had ever achieved through my own self-centered pursuits.

Another significant change was in how I approached my work. Instead of seeing it as a means to an end—a way to earn money, gain status, or prove my worth—I began to see it as an opportunity to express my values, to contribute to something larger than myself. I started to ask myself: How can I bring more authenticity, more integrity, and more passion into what I do? How can I use my skills, my knowledge, and my talents to make a positive impact in the world?

This shift in perspective transformed the way I experienced my work. It became less about what I could get from it and more about what I could give. I found that when I focused on serving others, on adding value, and on making a difference, I felt a deeper sense of satisfaction and fulfillment than I had ever felt before. I realized that success is not measured by what you achieve, but by how you contribute, how you connect, and how you grow.

One of the most liberating aspects of this journey was learning to let go of the need for perfection. For so long, I had believed that I needed to be perfect to be worthy—that I had to meet some impossible standard to be enough. But I began to see that perfection is an illusion, a trap that keeps you stuck in fear and self-doubt. I realized that real growth, real transformation, happens when you are willing to be imperfect, to make mistakes, to learn and to grow.

I learned to embrace my imperfections, to see them not as flaws but as opportunities for growth. I began to view my mistakes not as failures, but as valuable lessons that were helping me become a better, more compassionate, and more self-aware person. I discovered that it is in our imperfections that we find our greatest strengths—that our vulnerability, our humanity, is what makes us truly powerful.

As I continued to explore this new way of being, I found that my sense of purpose began to evolve. It became less about what I wanted to achieve or accomplish and more about how I wanted to live, how I wanted to show up in the world. I realized that purpose is not a destination but a direction—a way of moving through life with intention, with clarity, and with a deep sense of meaning.

I started to see that every moment, every choice, every action, is an opportunity to live with purpose. Whether it's how I choose to spend my time, how I treat the people around me, or how I respond to challenges and setbacks, I have the power to create a life that feels meaningful and fulfilling. I learned that purpose is not something that is handed to you; it is something you create, day by day, moment by moment, through the choices you make and the actions you take.

This journey from self-centeredness to self-awareness has been one of the most challenging and rewarding experiences of my life. It has required me to look deeply within, to confront my fears and insecurities, and to let go of the need for external validation. It has asked me to trust in myself, to believe in my own worth, and to have the courage to live in alignment with my values.

But it has also been incredibly liberating. It has given me a sense of peace and fulfillment that I never knew was possible. It has taught me that true happiness is not found in what you achieve or acquire, but in how you live, how you love, and how you give.

I have come to see that a purposeful life is not about being perfect or having it all figured out. It is about being true to yourself, about living with intention and integrity, and about finding joy in the journey, rather than in the destination. It is about embracing the messiness, the uncertainty, and the beauty of life, and about choosing, every day, to show up as the best version of yourself.

I am still on this journey. I am still learning, still growing, still discovering new facets of myself and new ways to live with purpose. But I am no longer afraid of the unknown. I am no longer chasing after something that always feels just out of reach. Instead, I am learning to find peace in the present moment, to trust in the process, and to embrace the adventure of becoming.

12.1 Finding Purpose: Aligning Actions with Values

Purpose, I've come to realize, is more than just a lofty goal or a distant destination. It's not something you chase after like a mirage on the horizon. Purpose is found in the alignment of what you do every day with the core of who you are. It's about finding harmony between your actions and your deepest values. This was a revelation that came to me slowly, almost painfully, over time. For years, I lived in a way that was completely detached from this understanding. I believed that purpose was about achieving greatness, about standing out, about making sure my voice was the loudest in the room. I thought that purpose was synonymous with success, with being admired and respected by others. But I was wrong.

When I started my journey toward self-awareness, the first step was to dig deep into what I truly valued. At first, this was an uncomfortable process. My values had been distorted by years of seeking approval, manipulating others, and clinging to a need for control. My old self would have listed things like power, recognition, and status as my top priorities. But as I started peeling back the layers, I discovered that these were not values at all. They were merely reflections of my insecurity, my fear of inadequacy, my desperate need to be seen.

So, I asked myself: What do I genuinely care about? What makes my soul feel alive? What gives me a sense of peace, of joy, of fulfillment? These were questions I had never truly considered before. And as I sat with them, I found myself returning to the simple things—kindness, compassion, connection, honesty. I realized that beneath all the noise, these were the things that truly mattered to me. They were the principles I wanted to build my life around.

But recognizing these values was only the beginning. The next challenge was to align my actions with them, to make sure that what I did each day was a reflection of what I believed in, what I stood for. This was harder than I imagined. It required a radical shift in the way I approached my life. It meant letting go of habits and behaviors that were deeply ingrained, that had defined me for so long. It meant stepping into a space of vulnerability, of uncertainty, of not knowing exactly what the outcome would be. But I knew it was necessary if I was ever going to find real purpose.

One of the first changes I made was to practice authenticity in every aspect of my life. For so long, I had worn a mask, presenting to the world a version of myself that I thought would be accepted, admired, and loved. I had hidden my true thoughts, my true feelings, for fear of rejection or judgment. But living inauthentically was exhausting. It kept me in a constant state of anxiety, always wondering if I was saying or doing the "right" thing.

So, I made a conscious decision to show up as myself, no matter the consequences. I began speaking my truth, expressing my real opinions, and sharing my genuine emotions. This wasn't easy. At times, it was terrifying. I worried that people wouldn't like the real me, that they would see my flaws, my imperfections, and turn away. But what I found was the opposite. The more I was honest about who I was, the more deeply I connected with others. I discovered that authenticity is magnetic; it draws people in, not because you're perfect, but because you're real.

Another critical step in aligning my actions with my values was to practice empathy in my interactions with others. I realized that for so long, I had been so focused on myself—my needs, my desires, my ambitions—that I had rarely stopped to consider how my actions affected those around me. I began to see that true empathy is not just about feeling for others; it's about actively choosing to put yourself in their shoes, to see the world from their perspective.

I started making a conscious effort to listen more deeply, to be fully present in my conversations, to ask questions, and to genuinely care about the answers. I learned to pause before reacting, to consider how my words and actions might impact the people I was speaking to. This was a practice that took time and patience, but it transformed my relationships in profound ways. I found that when I approached others with empathy and compassion, they responded with openness, trust, and vulnerability.

Aligning my actions with my values also meant finding ways to give back, to serve others in meaningful ways. I realized that purpose is not something you find in isolation, but in connection with the world around you. I started volunteering at local community centers, offering my time and resources to causes that resonated with me. I began mentoring individuals who were struggling with similar challenges, sharing my story, and offering support and guidance.

These experiences were eye-opening. They taught me that there is immense power in giving, in being of service, in contributing to something larger than yourself. They helped me see that purpose is not about what you achieve for yourself, but what you give to others. I found that in these moments of selfless service, I felt a sense of fulfillment and joy that I had never experienced before. It was a feeling that no amount of recognition or success could ever provide.

A significant aspect of this journey was learning to let go of the need for external validation. I realized that I had spent most of my life seeking approval from others, believing that my worth was tied to their opinions of me. But I began to see that true purpose comes from within, from knowing who you are and what you stand for, regardless of what others think. I started to trust myself more, to believe in my own instincts and judgments. I began to value my own voice, my own perspective, instead of constantly looking for affirmation from the outside world.

This was a radical shift for me, one that required a lot of self-reflection and inner work. But as I began to rely more on my inner compass, I found a newfound sense of freedom. I no longer felt the pressure to perform, to prove myself, to meet others' expectations. I realized that I was enough, just as I was, and that my purpose was not something I needed to earn or attain, but something I already had within me.

Another key component of aligning my actions with my values was practicing gratitude. I learned to cultivate a sense of appreciation for the present moment, for the small joys, the simple pleasures, the everyday miracles. I began to see that purpose is not something that exists in the future, but something that is created in the here and now. I learned to find joy in the process, in the journey, rather than in some distant outcome or goal.

Gratitude became a daily practice for me. Each morning, I would take a few moments to reflect on the things I was grateful for—the people in my life, the opportunities I had, the beauty of the world around me. I found that this practice shifted my perspective, helping me to see the abundance that already existed in my life, rather than focusing on what was lacking or missing. It helped me to live more mindfully, more intentionally, and to align my actions with a sense of purpose and meaning.

As I continued to explore this path, I also realized the importance of self-compassion. I had spent so much of my life being hard on myself, criticizing myself for my flaws, my mistakes, my perceived failures. But I began to see that true growth comes not from self-judgment, but from self-love. I learned to be kinder to myself, to forgive myself for my past, to recognize that I was doing the best I could with the knowledge and resources I had at the time.

Self-compassion became a cornerstone of my journey toward purpose. It allowed me to let go of the shame and guilt that had weighed me down for so long. It gave me the courage to take risks, to step out of my comfort zone, to pursue my passions and dreams, knowing that I would be okay no matter what the outcome. It taught me that my worth is not determined by my achievements, but by my capacity to love, to grow, and to be true to myself.

Ultimately, finding purpose and aligning my actions with my values has been about creating a life that feels authentic, meaningful, and true. It's about choosing, every day, to live in a way that reflects who I am at my core. It's about being intentional with my time, my energy, my resources, and making decisions that are in alignment with my beliefs and values.

This process is ongoing. It's a daily practice, a continuous journey of self-discovery and self-awareness. But it has brought me a sense of peace and fulfillment that I never knew was possible. It has taught me that purpose is not something you find in the world outside, but something you create within yourself. It is the act of living in alignment with your values, of being true to who you are, and of making a difference in the world in your own unique way.

Chapter 13: Helping Others Heal – Turning My Story into a Source of Strength

When I began this journey of self-awareness and transformation, I never imagined that my story would become a source of strength for others. In fact, for a long time, I didn't even want to share it. The shame of who I had been—the manipulations, the deceptions, the pain I caused—felt like a weight too heavy to bear, let alone expose to the world. But as I started to heal, I realized that there was power in sharing. I began to see that my story could be a light for others, a guide through the darkness of their own struggles.

I used to believe that the only way to help others was to be perfect, to present myself as someone who had it all together, who had never stumbled or fallen. But I have come to understand that perfection is not what inspires people; authenticity does. People don't connect with the flawless, the untouchable. They connect with the real, the vulnerable, the human. They find strength in the shared experience of our struggles, in the commonality of our pain and our joy.

So, I decided to be open about my journey, to let down my guard and show others the messy, imperfect process of my transformation. At first, it was terrifying. The fear of judgment, of rejection, of being misunderstood was overwhelming. But with every person who reached out to say, "Thank you for sharing your story—it made me feel less alone," I realized that this fear was a small price to pay for the impact I was making.

I began to speak publicly, to write about my experiences, to mentor others who were facing similar challenges. And what I found was that by helping others, I was continuing to heal myself. Every time I told my story, it felt like another layer of shame and guilt was being stripped away. I was reclaiming my narrative, taking ownership of my past, and using it as a tool for growth—for myself and for others.

One of the first steps I took was to become involved in support groups and communities that focused on healing from narcissistic abuse. These were spaces where people came together to share their experiences, to offer each other support and understanding. At first, I simply listened. I wanted to hear other people's stories, to learn from their experiences, to understand their pain. It was a humbling experience. I heard stories that broke my heart—stories of betrayal, of manipulation, of deep emotional wounds. But I also heard stories of incredible resilience, of strength, of hope.

Gradually, I began to share my own story in these spaces. I was honest about my past, about the ways I had hurt others, about the long road I had traveled to come to terms with who I had been. I spoke about the moments of despair, the nights when I lay awake, haunted by the things I had done, the people I had hurt. And I spoke about the breakthroughs, the moments of clarity, the small victories along the way.

To my surprise, people responded with empathy, with compassion, with gratitude. Many of them had encountered narcissists in their own lives, and they appreciated hearing from someone who was on the other side of that behavior, who was trying to change. They asked me questions about my journey, about what had helped me, about the tools and strategies I had used to change my behavior.

These conversations were incredibly healing for me. They helped me to see that I was not alone in my struggle, that there were others out there who were also trying to navigate this complex path of self-awareness and growth. They also made me realize that I had something valuable to offer, that my experiences could serve as a guide for others who were on a similar journey.

Over time, I began to take a more active role in these communities. I volunteered to facilitate group discussions, to lead workshops on healing and self-awareness. I drew from my own experiences, from the lessons I had learned, from the mistakes I had made. I spoke about the importance of empathy, of self-reflection, of taking responsibility for one's actions. I shared practical tools for self-growth, like journaling, mindfulness practices, and communication skills.

I found that people were hungry for this kind of guidance. Many of them had been dealing with narcissists for years, and they were desperate for a way out, for a path to healing. They wanted to know how to protect themselves, how to set boundaries, how to rebuild their self-esteem. And I realized that I had the answers—not because I was an expert, but because I had been there. I had lived it. I had made the mistakes, and I had learned from them.

I began to see that my story was not just about me; it was about all of us. It was about the shared experience of pain and healing, of falling down and getting back up, of being lost and finding our way. It was about the human capacity for growth, for change, for redemption. And I wanted to use my story to show others that this was possible—that no matter how far you had fallen, no matter how much damage you had caused, there was always a way back. There was always a way to make things right, to become the person you were meant to be.

I also realized that helping others was a way for me to continue my own growth. Every time I offered support to someone else, every time I listened to their story, I was reminded of the importance of empathy, of compassion, of understanding. I was reminded that we are all in this together, that we are all struggling in our own ways, and that we all have the capacity to heal, to grow, to change.

In mentoring others, I found a new purpose, a new sense of meaning in my life. I discovered that my past, with all its mistakes and regrets, could be transformed into something positive, something that could make a difference in the lives of others. I found that by helping others to heal, I was continuing to heal myself.

One of the most powerful moments of my journey was when I started to receive messages from people who had read my story or attended one of my talks. They told me how my words had resonated with them, how they had seen themselves in my story, how they had found hope in my journey. Some of them were people who had been hurt by narcissists; others were people who, like me, had struggled with narcissistic traits themselves. They shared their own stories with me—their struggles, their pain, their victories.

These messages were incredibly moving. They made me realize that my story was having a real impact, that it was helping people in a way I had never imagined. It was giving them permission to be imperfect, to make mistakes, to struggle, and to grow. It was showing them that healing is possible, that change is possible, that there is always a way forward.

I also began to work one-on-one with individuals who were trying to heal from narcissistic abuse or who were grappling with their own narcissistic tendencies. I found that my unique perspective—having been on both sides of the equation—was incredibly valuable. I could speak to the pain of being hurt by a narcissist, but I could also speak to the pain of being the narcissist, of living with that behavior, of trying to change it.

I found that people appreciated this dual perspective. They felt seen, understood, validated. They felt like they were not alone in their struggles, that there was someone who truly understood what they were going through. And I found that by sharing my experiences, by being open and honest about my journey, I was able to build trust, to create a safe space for them to open up, to explore their own emotions, their own experiences, their own paths to healing.

Through this process, I learned that helping others is not about having all the answers; it's about being willing to show up, to be present, to listen, to care. It's about being willing to share your own story, not as a blueprint for someone else's journey, but as a source of inspiration, a reminder that they are not alone, that they are not broken, that they are not beyond repair.

I also learned that there is immense power in community. Healing is not something you do in isolation; it's something you do together. It's about finding people who understand, who empathize, who support you, who hold you accountable. It's about building connections, creating networks of support, finding strength in the collective.

Today, I am committed to using my story to help others heal. I am committed to being a voice for those who are struggling, who are lost, who are in pain. I am committed to showing them that there is always a way forward, that there is always hope, that they are not alone.

I know that I still have a lot to learn, that I am still growing, still healing, still finding my way. But I also know that my journey is not just about me; it's about all of us. It's about the shared human experience of pain and healing, of struggle and growth, of falling down and getting back up. And I am grateful every day for the opportunity to share my story, to use my experiences as a source of strength, to help others find their own path to healing.

13.1 Mentoring and Coaching: Supporting Others on Their Journey

Mentoring and coaching others who are on their path to healing has become one of the most rewarding aspects of my transformation. After years of working through my own issues, confronting my past behaviors, and learning to embrace vulnerability, I've realized that there is immense value in guiding others through their journeys. It's a privilege and a responsibility I take seriously, understanding the profound impact that shared experiences and encouragement can have on someone's growth.

My decision to step into a mentoring role didn't happen overnight. It was a gradual realization that my story and the hard lessons I've learned could provide others with the support and insight they might need. There was a time when I questioned whether I was truly capable of helping others. After all, I had once been a narcissist—the person who caused pain rather than healed it. But as I began to see the changes in my own life, I realized that my unique perspective could serve as a beacon for those lost in the darkness of similar struggles. I understood their pain because I had been both the perpetrator and the reformer. I knew their fears, their doubts, and their hopes, because I had lived through them.

One of the first steps I took in this direction was to reach out to people in online communities and local support groups where individuals were seeking help, guidance, or just a sympathetic ear. I started small, offering to listen, to share my own experiences, and to provide practical advice. I quickly realized how desperate people were for understanding, for someone who could relate to their experiences without judgment. There was an overwhelming need for empathy, validation, and support—things that I had also craved during my journey. I became aware that many people felt isolated and overwhelmed, unsure of where to turn or how to begin healing.

In these initial interactions, I made a conscious effort to approach each conversation with genuine curiosity and compassion. I listened deeply, aware that sometimes, people simply needed to be heard. I didn't pretend to have all the answers, nor did I try to fix everything in a single conversation. Instead, I focused on being present, on holding space for others to explore their emotions, their thoughts, and their fears. This was a crucial lesson for me: that mentoring wasn't about giving advice from a pedestal, but rather about walking alongside someone as they navigated their own path.

As I became more comfortable in this role, I realized that many people needed not just empathy but also practical strategies for navigating their challenges. They needed tools for coping with anxiety, for setting boundaries, for managing their emotions, and for building healthier relationships. Drawing from my own experience, I began to develop a more structured approach to mentoring. I started offering personalized coaching sessions, where I could work one-on-one with individuals to help them identify their goals, understand their obstacles, and develop actionable steps toward healing.

These coaching sessions often began with the question: "What do you hope to achieve?" It was a simple question, but it often opened the door to profound conversations about fear, hope, and resilience. Some wanted to break free from toxic relationships, others wanted to heal from childhood trauma, and still others sought to understand and change their own harmful behaviors. By helping them articulate their goals, I found that I could help them see a path forward, even if that path was still shrouded in uncertainty.

In these sessions, I emphasized the importance of self-reflection, self-awareness, and self-compassion—three pillars that had been instrumental in my own journey. I encouraged my clients to keep journals, to write down their thoughts and feelings, to explore their emotional responses to different situations, and to track their progress over time. This practice of reflection helped them become more aware of their patterns, more attuned to their triggers, and more compassionate toward themselves. It also gave them a tangible way to see their growth, which was incredibly motivating.

Another critical aspect of my mentoring approach was helping others build resilience. I had learned through my own journey that setbacks were inevitable, but they didn't have to be the end of the story. Resilience, I taught them, wasn't about never falling down; it was about learning how to get back up again. I helped them identify their strengths, their sources of support, and their coping mechanisms. I encouraged them to practice self-care, to build routines that nurtured their physical, emotional, and mental well-being, and to celebrate their small victories along the way.

I also found it important to create a safe space where my clients could express their feelings without fear of judgment. Many of them carried deep shame, anger, or grief, and they needed to know that it was okay to feel these emotions. I reassured them that healing wasn't a linear process, that it was okay to have good days and bad days, to take two steps forward and one step back. I reminded them that growth often comes from the messiest, most uncomfortable places, and that it was okay to be a work in progress.

In my role as a mentor, I also recognized the importance of modeling vulnerability. I shared my own stories of failure and struggle, my moments of doubt and fear, my challenges in changing old patterns and building new ones. I was honest about my own imperfections, my ongoing work to be better, and my commitment to living a more authentic life. This openness helped to build trust and connection, to show my clients that they were not alone, and to remind them that it was okay to be imperfect.

One of the most transformative experiences I've had as a mentor was working with a client who was struggling with her own narcissistic tendencies. She was a successful professional, highly driven, and charismatic, but she had begun to notice how her behavior was pushing people away, how her relationships were suffering. She was scared, confused, and didn't know where to begin. In our first session, she admitted that she had never been able to connect with others on a deep emotional level. She confessed that she often felt empty, isolated, and consumed by a need for validation and control.

Together, we began to unpack her fears, her insecurities, and her past experiences that had shaped her current behavior. We talked about her childhood, her relationships, her career, and her patterns of thinking. I helped her see that her narcissistic traits were not a fixed part of her identity, but rather learned behaviors that could be changed with effort and commitment. I encouraged her to take small steps toward vulnerability, to practice empathy, and to challenge her need for control.

Over time, she began to open up, to share her emotions more freely, to ask for help, to apologize when she hurt others, and to build more authentic connections. She also started to see herself in a different light—not as a monster, but as a human being who was capable of change. Watching her transformation was one of the most rewarding experiences of my life. It was a powerful reminder that change is possible, that healing is possible, and that we are all capable of growth.

Throughout my mentoring journey, I have learned that each person's path is unique. There is no one-size-fits-all approach to healing. What works for one person may not work for another. That's why I always try to tailor my approach to the individual, to meet them where they are, to understand their unique needs, strengths, and challenges. I don't pretend to have all the answers, but I do promise to walk alongside them, to support them, to cheer them on, and to help them find their way.

My goal as a mentor is not to fix people, but to empower them. I want to help them see their own potential, to recognize their own worth, to understand that they are not defined by their past, but by the choices they make today. I want to help them build the skills, the habits, and the mindset they need to create a better future for themselves and for the people they care about.

I also believe that mentoring is a two-way street. While I strive to help others, I am constantly learning from them as well. Each person I work with teaches me something new about resilience, about courage, about the human spirit. They remind me of the power of vulnerability, of empathy, of connection. They inspire me to keep growing, to keep learning, to keep striving to be a better version of myself.

Ultimately, mentoring is not just about helping others; it's about building a community of support, of understanding, of compassion. It's about creating a space where people can come together to share their stories, to heal their wounds, to celebrate their victories, and to support each other on their journeys. It's about reminding each other that we are not alone, that we are stronger together, and that no matter how dark things may seem, there is always a way forward.

By mentoring and coaching others, I've found a deeper purpose in my own life. I've discovered that my past, with all its mistakes and regrets, has value—not just for me, but for others as well. I've learned that by sharing my story, by offering my support, by being present and engaged, I can make a difference. I can help others heal. And in doing so, I continue to heal myself.

Mentoring has become a vital part of my own growth, a way to stay accountable, to stay humble, and to stay connected. It has taught me that true strength lies not in perfection, but in the willingness to be vulnerable, to be open, to be human. It has shown me that by lifting others up, we lift ourselves up as well. And it has reminded me that no matter where we come from, no matter what we've done, we all have the capacity to change, to grow, and to become the best versions of ourselves.

In mentoring others, I have found not just a way to give back, but a way to keep moving forward, a way to keep living with purpose, with intention, and with hope.

Conclusion: The Final Journal – A Narrative of Redemption and Peace

As I sit here, pen in hand, reflecting on this long and often painful journey, I am struck by the paradox of it all. The beginning seems like a distant, almost surreal chapter of someone else's life. I was lost in a world shaped by ego, entitlement, and a desperate need for validation. I used manipulation like a tool, wielded control like a weapon, and justified my actions with a twisted sense of self-righteousness. I was the narcissist, trapped in my own web of deceit, yet blind to the reality of my own behavior.

I remember the first time I allowed myself to truly see. It wasn't a dramatic moment, but rather a quiet realization that settled over me like a heavy fog. It began with a gnawing discomfort, a sense that something wasn't quite right. I dismissed it at first, pushing it aside as I had always done with emotions that threatened my carefully constructed reality. But the feeling persisted, growing louder and more insistent until I could no longer ignore it. It was as if a small crack had formed in the walls of my fortress, letting in a thin, piercing beam of light.

That light was self-awareness. It wasn't sudden or overwhelming, but gradual and unnerving. I began to see myself not as the victim or the misunderstood hero, but as someone capable of causing harm. I saw the hurt in the eyes of those I loved, the distance I had created between myself and the world, the isolation that came not from others but from within me. The walls I had built to protect myself had, in fact, become my prison.

In the quiet moments of reflection, I started to understand the depth of the damage I had caused. I saw the ripple effect of my actions, how each lie, each manipulation, each act of selfishness had created waves that reached far beyond my own small world. I saw the faces of those I had hurt, the trust I had shattered, the love I had twisted into something unrecognizable. It was a hard truth to face, but it was the beginning of my redemption.

The path to healing was not a straight line; it was a winding road filled with setbacks and breakthroughs. I had to unlearn so much of what I had thought to be true. I had to confront the parts of myself that I had spent years avoiding. I had to face the reality that I was not the person I had believed myself to be. I was not the victim, nor was I the hero. I was just a person, flawed and human, trying to navigate a world that I had misunderstood for so long.

Final Journal Entry

I woke up this morning with a lightness I hadn't felt in years. It was one of those moments that seemed almost ordinary, yet carried with it a sense of profound peace. I could hear the birds outside my window, the soft rustle of leaves in the wind, the distant hum of the world waking up. For so long, I had been at war with myself — fighting against the person I was, battling with the person I wanted to become. But today, there was no battle. Just a quiet acceptance, a deep understanding that I am finally okay.

I sat down with my journal, a habit I had formed in the depths of my struggle to find myself. The words flowed more freely now, no longer tangled with guilt or fear. I wrote about the changes I've seen in myself, the way I've started to notice the small things, the little moments that bring joy. I wrote about the friends I've made, real friends who see me for who I am, not for who I pretend to be. I wrote about my family, the healing that has taken place, the bridges slowly being rebuilt, one honest conversation at a time.

I wrote about my mistakes, not with shame, but with a sense of gratitude. Every wrong turn, every hurtful word, every manipulative game — they were all lessons, paths that led me here, to this moment of clarity. I realized that my journey wasn't just about becoming less narcissistic; it was about becoming more human. It was about embracing all parts of myself, even the broken ones, and finding strength in that vulnerability.

Today, I feel free. Not in the way I once thought freedom meant — power, control, superiority — but free in the truest sense of the word. Free to be myself, to make mistakes, to be imperfect. Free to love and be loved, not for what I can give, but for who I am. Free to live a life that feels right, that feels true to me.

I know I am still a work in progress. I know there will be days when doubt creeps in, when old habits try to reassert themselves, when I feel tempted to slip back into the shadows. But I also know that I have the tools, the awareness, and the courage to face those moments. I know I have grown, and I know I will keep growing.

I closed my journal and felt a tear slide down my cheek — not a tear of sadness, but of relief, of release. I am not the person I used to be, but I am also not yet the person I will become. I am somewhere in between, and for the first time, I am okay with that. I am okay with the uncertainty, the unknown, the process of becoming.

As I head into the day, I feel a quiet confidence, a calm assurance that no matter what happens, I am enough. I have found my way out of the darkness, not by fighting it, but by embracing the light within. And that is a journey worth taking, a story worth telling, a life worth living.

Reflecting on the entire journey, I realize it was never about reaching some perfect end state. It was about learning to live in the present, with all its messiness and uncertainty, and finding peace in that. I understand now that I cannot erase my past, but I can choose to learn from it. I can choose to make amends, to rebuild trust, to offer love and understanding where once there was only judgment and control.

Learning to empathize with others was transformative. I began to see people not as extensions of my own needs and desires, but as individuals with their own stories, pain, and worth. I listened more, spoke less, and felt with them, not just for them. It was humbling, and it opened my heart in ways I never thought possible. I realized empathy is not a skill to master, but a way of being, a daily choice to step outside oneself and truly connect.

Building new habits took time. I replaced manipulation with honesty, fear with courage, and isolation with connection. I practiced kindness, not just towards others, but also toward myself. I allowed myself to be imperfect, to make mistakes, to fall and get back up. I began to trust in the process, in the slow, steady growth that comes from consistent effort and genuine intention.

Forgiving myself was perhaps the hardest part. I had to let go of the shame and guilt that kept me chained to my past. I realized that forgiveness was not about condoning my behavior, but about freeing myself to move forward. It was about understanding that I am not defined by my worst moments, but by my capacity to change, to grow, to become someone better.

This journey has taught me that life is not about avoiding pain or seeking perfection, but about finding meaning in the struggle, purpose in the process, and joy in the small, everyday moments of connection and growth. I have learned that true freedom comes not from control, but from letting go. That true strength lies not in power, but in vulnerability. And that true love is not about possession, but about acceptance, understanding, and empathy.

I am grateful for this journey, for every step, every stumble, every breakthrough. I am grateful for the people who stood by me, for those who challenged me, and even for those who walked away. They all taught me something, and they all played a part in my transformation.

So here I am, no longer the narcissist, but a human being, flawed and beautiful, striving every day to be better than I was the day before. I have found peace, not in perfection, but in authenticity. I have found joy, not in control, but in connection. And I have found love, not in manipulation, but in genuine, heartfelt empathy.

This is my story, my journey out of narcissism. A journey from chaos to clarity, from darkness to light, from fear to love. And for that, I am profoundly, eternally grateful.

My greatest wish for you is that, like me, you find your way back to living fully. May you embrace the lessons learned, forgive yourself for past mistakes, and step into the future with courage and compassion. This book was not just a personal reflection but also a way to reach out to others who may be struggling. We all have the capacity to change, to grow, and to heal.
Thank you for allowing me to be a part of your journey, and I hope that you, too, can rediscover the joy, peace, and fulfillment that comes with living in truth and love.
With sincere gratitude and hope.

Katashi Yoshimura

Printed in Great Britain
by Amazon